MEN, LOVE & BIRTH

MEN, LOVE & BIRTH

The book about being present at birth
that your pregnant lover wants you to read

pinter & martin

Men, Love & Birth: the book about being present at birth that your pregnant lover wants you to read

First published by Pinter & Martin Ltd 2015
reprinted 2015, 2017

Text copyright © Mark Harris 2015

Illustrations copyright © Jon Lander 2015

Mark Harris has asserted his moral rights to be identified as the author of this work in accordance with the Copyright, Designs and Patents Act of 1988.

Text in appendix 2 © Katie Whitehouse, reprinted by kind permission of the author

Photographs in appendix 2 © Kate Mount

Author photograph Martin Neeves Photography & Film

ISBN 978-1-78066-225-1
Also available as ebook

British Library Cataloguing-in-Publication Data
A catalogue record for this book is available from the British Library.

Printed and bound in the EU by Hussar

Pinter & Martin Ltd
6 Effra Parade
London SW2 1PS

pinterandmartin.com

To my Gorgeeeeee
'We found love in a hopeless place'

CONTENTS

FOREWORD

Men, Love & Birth is a unique contribution to the literature on contemporary childbirth because it speaks into the experience of tens of thousands of men who now accompany their partners for the labour and birth event. The expectation that male partners should be at the birth is almost routine in many high-income countries. And, like many other practices around childbirth, the benefits or disadvantages of this practice are unknown, at least from a research perspective. This is of little comfort to the many men who have trod this path, usually with some trepidation, as the expectation that they are there has become culturally embedded. At last there is a book written just for them, and no one is better qualified to write it than Mark Harris. He has the important advantage of seeing this experience from both sides of the fence – as a father of six children and as a midwife, working within the NHS for a number of years.

Mark's style is direct, candid and self-disclosing, distilling an incredible breadth of reading and experience into punchy, accessible chapters that range over in-depth childbirth physiology through to love-making positions for pregnancy and of course labour and birth itself. Prepare to be amused, informed, challenged and moved by his self-deprecating anecdotes and colloquial language. Mark achieves the tricky balance of explaining complicated theories and ideas in a straightforward way and then offers practical tasks and exercises to apply them to real life. He draws on a range of theorists and theories in building an approach to birth that seeks to maximise women's potential to birth safely and healthily. For most women, that will mean natural, normal birth. His midwifery lens shines through everything he writes and he is therefore able to demystify the terminology of labour that can obscure a fundamentally physiological process.

He introduces the concept of male and female energies that both men and women possess and describes how men can channel those energies for the benefit of their partner, illustrating this with lots of practical tips and advice. Building on his interactions with many men through his Birthing For Blokes website and workshops, he details a typical workshop discussion towards the end of the book that captures much of his teaching in extended conversational extracts.

This book is intended to help men engage in a positive way with an experience outside of their comfort zone that, let's face it, has the potential to be upsetting for them and counterproductive for their partners. But by understanding the purpose behind evolutionary processes and how birth hormones work, we can change that dynamic so that it is exciting and rewarding for them and enabling for the one they love. It may even help to change the way we manage birth in the twenty-first century and rescue it from unnecessary medicalisation, something midwife researchers like me and my colleagues have been trying to address for decades.

Denis Walsh
Associate Professor in Midwifery
Nottingham University

INTRODUCTION

People always struggle to guess what I do for a living. I've won more than one round of drinks playing that game. When I finally reveal, three pints later, that I'm a midwife, people still don't believe it.

It's not much different when I'm at work. I walk into the birth room and the woman says, 'I called the midwife, not security', to which I reply, 'I am the midwife'. She then shouts, 'SECURITY'!

I do understand that response. Imagine your partner is in the throes of the birthing process, just about managing the intensity of the uterine tightenings, and in walks a 20 stone, shaven-headed, biker-looking bloke doing jazz hands. (I do my best not to do the hands thing, but it's become a bit of a habit).

When I first started out as a student midwife, there were only 61 male midwives out of 36,000 in the whole of the UK. I remember standing at the foot of a woman's bed, having been asked by my mentor to do my first vaginal examination. My mind was racing, and more than a little panicked, I thought, 'Please, please let this not be the first time I stumble on the clitoris!'

I am often asked why I became a midwife, given how unusual it is for a man to do the job. I do come from a large family – five sisters and three brothers – and now I have six children and six grandchildren. Maybe this is what has created a love of pregnancy and birth in me? It does mean that my contraceptive advice is probably crap.

My sons grew up in a household where a man being a midwife was normal. In fact they wanted to be midwives like their dad until they realised that being a midwife was considered a 'woman's job'. Then, when their friends asked them what their dad did for a living, they would say, 'Oh, nothing, he's unemployed'.

My mother left an indelible mark on me: she gave birth to eight children with little medical help. After having her last child aged 46, she went on to adopt a child too. In many ways I have followed in her footsteps, gaining a deep faith in a woman's inner power to give birth.

It's impossible to underestimate the power of a mother and father's influence on a young child's developing personality. My mum teased me mercilessly about my weight. For as long as I can remember I have struggled to lose weight and have been self-conscious about my size. She used to say that my first school photograph was an aerial shot, and that she took me to school in a wheelbarrow. (A little harsh, methinks.)

Being a male midwife is one thing; looking like an extra

from *Gangs of New York* is another. I did look after one woman, who once she had calmed down after the birth said to me that I looked like an actor. 'Oh,' she said, 'You know – it's on the tip of my tongue.' I was thinking, an overweight Vin Diesel? Or a plump Bruce Willis? Finally, she got it. 'SHREK!' she exclaimed.

My mental battle with size was brought into sharp focus when, not long after joining a new midwifery team, I was invited on one of those 'Outward Bound' team-building days. All the others had done their abseil down the side of a bridge. It was a long way down, and I was more than nervous. 'Has that rope got a weight limit?' I asked. 'You'd get a minibus on this rope', the weathered instructor said, encouragingly. By now I was properly scared, desperate to get out of doing it without losing face. 'Have you ever had a minibus on it?' I asked, wanting to keep the conversation going as long as I could. 'Nope', he said, 'You're the closest we've come'!

My weight has never stopped me from playing sports: cricket, football, rugby, and tennis, anything with a ball really. These skills have come in use at least once in my midwifery career. I was once looking after a woman having her seventh baby. She chose to birth standing up, a position that makes perfect sense from an anatomical and gravitational perspective, which makes birth easier.

Given it was her baby number seven (all born vaginally), she could probably have given birth while doing a handstand. She stood, rocked and then gave birth to her baby. He shot out and I had to dive to my left like a fielder in the slips to catch him. I resisted the urge to throw him in the air shouting 'Howzat?!'

I have been registered as a midwife since 1994 and as a nurse since 1991. I love being around people and this has influenced the choices I have made in my professional life. In addition to my midwifery training I have trained and worked as a teacher in further education, hypnotherapist, NLP (neuro linguistic programme) trainer, outreach youth worker and nurse in a secure mental health rehab unit. I still work as a midwife, offering birth education through a programme called Birthing For Blokes*. Work and play often merge for me.

Why did I decide to run birth preparation classes for men? I knew there was already at least one company providing education and birth preparation classes for men, and I was undecided about the benefits of it. I remember mentioning the idea on Facebook. One of my midwife friends felt very strongly that there was no need for it, and that any focus on a man in this context was time wasted. My time, she felt, would be better invested in being with the woman. She makes a good point, particularly when midwives in hospital are hard pressed to find the time to be intensely focused on a woman's needs, and are pulled in many directions, often looking after more than one woman while also being asked to complete a never-ending pile of paperwork.

---

* birthing4blokes.com

Nevertheless, I decided to run some experimental classes for men whose partners were pregnant. The more I thought about it, the more I felt there was something unique that I could offer these men. In over 20 years as a qualified midwife, my observations of how men respond to the intensity of the emotions in the birth room, generated by the hormones released into their bloodstream as birthing takes place, has taught me a lot. Being present at birth provokes a wide range of behaviour in men, from angry, confrontational shouting, to becoming withdrawn and playing games on a tablet.

The decision to start the Birthing For Blokes workshop sessions was profoundly influenced by the death of my wife of 20 years, Diane. She died from cancer on 19 March 2008, the day before my birthday. As I was registering her death I knew that my life would never be the same; I resolved then that I would only ever do work that I wanted to do, that I felt made a distinctive difference to the lives of others.

The day after my birthday I woke to a colourless world. My life had been ransacked. I was responsible for five children. Home-schooling, providing for them and doing my best to love enough for two people more than occupied my time. Through tears I remember how desperately bleak the future looked then, but bad as things were I knew they would get better. My new-found determination to share what I had learnt from my experiences of being around men as their lovers gave birth would give direction to my future plans.

I left my regular paying job in the NHS and started to work for myself. There was no money coming in unless I created it. I was afraid of not being able to pay direct debits, but amazingly liberated from that horrible feeling of not wanting to go to work, of dreading working with others who seemed so overwhelmingly bland and hamstrung by the way they had always thought. In the main the 'caring types' I have worked with over the years have meant well, but the demands of the organisations they work for, and the sheer volume of people they need to see, have worn them down.

I now ensure that all I do is completely down to choice. Of course I've always had a choice, it's just never really felt like it. When the children started to arrive I always felt that I had to work, and leaving a job with nothing else to do was unthinkable. Yet looking back, some years on, surrounded by grandchildren and another beautiful child of my own, with a wonderful partner by my side, it's hard to believe that life is so different.

I met Trez in a pub by accident. I was learning lines for a little theatre play I had been cast in, slowly getting drunk over my Guinness – which was probably the only reason I had the courage to ask for her number. I feel enormously grateful to have met a woman who knows me as she does, yet offers the kind of unconditional love that requires no change in me.

why have I written this book?

Having been a midwife for 20 years and a man for longer, I have experience that I know is useful. I have insights that will help both first-time fathers and those becoming fathers again. Being both a man and a midwife has helped me to realise that, as a man, I have to yield to a woman's innate knowing when she births. The powerful dance of the feminine cannot be resisted; learning to dance with her is what this book is all about.

Blokes have often said to me, 'I felt left out, I didn't know what was going on, I felt powerless'. That feeling of not being able to do anything to protect your partner when she needs you most can be too much for many men. When the woman you love is crying out, as the intensity of the birthing process takes her close to the edge of panic, being told to 'calm down', or worse, 'stay out of the way', is guaranteed to generate huge amounts of adrenaline in you. This hormone has evolved over generations to create the energy for a 'fight', to equip you as a warrior, ready to protect your lover from predators. It can be difficult to handle in the modern-day birth context: the 'predators' you now need to protect her from are not wild beasts, but the feelings of fear that will slow the birthing process down.

I have found over the years that an understanding of how evolutionary forces have shaped our responses to the birthing process as human beings is often all we really need to help us discover the brilliance that lies inside ourselves as men, a brilliance that has been tried and tested over 200,000 years or so of human existence.

I hope to put the prospect of imminent fatherhood in the context of being a man, and explore how your presence at the birth of your child can be a rite of passage. Our culture has lost many of these 'coming of age' rituals, although they survive among indigenous groups elsewhere in the world. They can be powerful, almost theatrical ceremonies, in which boys become men. Women, of course, have physiologically in-built 'rites of passage': periods (girl–woman), and birth (woman–mother). But what 'rites of passage' do men have in modern society? Our voices break, we grow facial hair and we might play a few risky games on the PlayStation! Birth, for a bloke, can be a rite of passage too. When it is, a MAN does the fathering! It feels a little cheesy to talk about blokes becoming warriors. I don't mean fighters, or violent types, I mean strong MEN who are able to manage life and fatherhood.

I love being a father. Watching my children grow, change and mature as they experience life is never boring and often exhilarating. Fatherhood, when built upon the warrior-like support you give the woman you love as she gives birth, provides a foundation of tender-hearted strength. A solid base helps build the kind of strength needed for good fathering to take place in the future.

who is this book for?

This is primarily a book for men who are about to become fathers. I want to prepare you by giving you an understanding of the environments that are truly supportive of 'good birth'. I mean both a woman's internal environment (a quiet mind), and her external environment, the place where she is to give birth (a quiet place).

Too many men I have been with in the birth room over the years have left it with mixed emotions. Often they feel very tired, both physically and mentally. Of course they are elated – witnessing the birth of your baby will be a profound experience – but these feelings of elation may be tempered by a sense of regret or shame at not being able to 'do anything' when the woman they loved seemed to need them most.

By reading this book and doing the exercises, both on your own and with your partner, you give yourself the best chance of being ready when the whirlwind of the birthing process takes hold of her. You will be able to create a safe space for her, so that she can 'lose' herself in the ancient rhythms of birth that have served birthing women for countless generations. Your task is to facilitate in her the development of a quiet mind, and in the external world a quiet place for the birth of your family to unfold. The rest of this book will help you discover the inner resources that you and your lover already possess.

Having read this book you will:

from Chapter 1

- Learn how evolution has worked to make you and your lover perfectly equipped to experience the birth of your baby.
- Achieve an understanding of what is happening to her throughout the birthing process. This wisdom will enable you to offer the support she needs when she needs it.
- Learn how your body works in the birth situation: this will give you a head start in managing your fight, flight or freeze response.
- Create an action plan of ways that you can create a quiet environment best suited for fantastic birth.

from Chapter 2

- Be reminded that men and women are different not just anatomically, but emotionally and spiritually.
- Begin to notice how all human beings have both masculine and feminine energy regardless of their gender, and how these energies are lived out on a day-to-day basis.
- Discover how knowing about the expression of feminine and masculine energy influences your relationship, your sex life and the kind of birth your lover will experience.
- Discover the power that is released in your life as you learn to become fully present to your lover as an expression of your masculine energy.

- Have a sense of how you being present as she gives birth can act as a kind of initiation ritual, becoming a powerful stimulus to being a father.
- Learn exercises that will lead you into this sense of presence at will, which will prepare you for being fully present as she gives birth.

from Chapter 3

- Have an understanding of how human beings are 'meaning-making machines'.
- Learn a new model of communication, through which you can make sense of the world. The ways in which you construct internal mental maps, based on the five senses, which you use to make sense of the enormous amounts of raw data received every second.
- Know ways in which this new knowledge regarding communication can be applied to create a quiet mind in your lover.
- Have a new appreciation for the work that your unconscious mind, and your partner's does to keep your bodies and lives working well, particularly during the birthing process.
- Have an appreciation of the limits of your conscious mind and the vast resources that your unconscious mind possesses.
- Learn exercises and practices that enable you to unleash the power of your unconscious mind, better enabling you to serve your pregnant lover and prepare you for fatherhood.

- Have an understanding of how language is learned and processed unconsciously and the power of language to direct our meaning-making and that of others.
- Be able to break the 'curses and spells' that health professionals unwittingly cast upon your pregnant lover, casting your own spells designed to create a quiet mind in her.

from Chapters 4, 5 & 6

- Have answers to some of the most important questions posed by your lover's imminent birth. Talking about these choices and making decisions should be done long before the birthing process starts. Some of those questions might be:
  - Is home birth safe?
  - What can I do if we want a home birth but our doctor or midwife is saying no?
  - What is the best position for the baby to be in before the birthing process starts and how can you help to make that happen?
  - What causes the birthing process to start?
  - How do you know that the birthing process has started?
  - What are the stages of the birthing process, and how will you know she is progressing well?
  - How will you know your baby is well, before the birthing process starts and through the birthing process?
  - What do doctors mean when they say your

partner is 'overdue'?

- What does 'induction of labour' mean? If it's going to happen to your lover, how might it be done?
- If your lover is finding the uterine tightenings difficult to manage, what is available to help her with them?
- How can your partner use different postures and body positions to facilitate the birthing process?

from Chapter 7

· How breastfeeding works and why it is important.
· How you can support your partner effectively.
· Why your role is important.

1
BIRTH FROM AN EVOLUTIONARY PERSPECTIVE

Evolution is no slouch. We come from a long line of successfully birthing women! You and I are living proof that the birthing process works perfectly. If it didn't, we wouldn't be here. It's that simple. Women have a 200,000-year history of birthing well; men have only been present at birth for about fifty of those years. Evolutionary biologists tell us that changes to biological systems take many, many generations: this means that we effectively have Stone Age bodies now living in the fast lane of modern life. Our physiological responses are ancient, and adapted to a different context than the one we find ourselves in today.

From an evolutionary point of view, and looking at the biological and hormonal adaptations of human beings, the part of the brain responsible for a woman birthing well is the limbic system. This part of the brain is a lot older than the neocortex and has many functions, but the ones of interest in our discussion are those responsible for 'thinking' and 'meaning-making': human beings are meaning-making machines. It's the very act that marks us out as different from other animals. We can produce language and we have the ability to think about thinking.

The limbic system is the mammalian part of the brain. When a woman who is giving birth is able to lose herself in the work of this ancient system, which is responsible for the hormones that start and keep the birthing process going, and when the thinking work of the neocortex is turned off, she is simply a mammal birthing, an animal responding instinctively. No meaning-making (talking, thinking) is required to make the birth of her baby successful.

As Fritz Perls (1893–1970), a German-born psychiatrist and psychologist, said: she needs to 'lose her mind and come to her sense'. Your job, as her lover, is to be fully present, and through your presence to create a safe space in which she can truly let go. The next chapter will talk more about this.

When you understand the power that generations of evolutionary development have had over the birthing process, you can begin to develop a deep sense of faith. Knowing that birth works well, and has done so for a long time, means that you can begin to relax.

We live in a society where doctors habitually try to convince women and their partners that they need them in order for birth to happen safely. Over the years birth has been medicalised and defined by 'risk'. Men regularly tell me that they are afraid of the prospect of their partner giving birth, and if their partner wants a home birth, for example, that fear comes to the fore, often in defensive ways.

Your evolution as a man has given you what you need to be with her as she gives birth. An understanding of what is going on in your body and hers is one of the keys to truly loving the experience and being the very best you can be in the situation.

what happens for her?

As the birthing process starts for a woman, the ancient parts of her brain (the limbic system) are releasing oxytocin, and a mix of other hormones. Oxytocin is a powerful hormone, responsible for keeping the process moving forward, climaxing in the birth of a new human being.

The structures of a woman's brain responsible for the release of oxytocin do not respond well to 'thinking'. They cannot be talked into working well. A woman in the midst of birthing will enter into an altered state of awareness, which enhances her unconscious ability to bathe her body in the 'hormone sea' needed for rewarding birth to take place.

The neocortex's ability to 'think about thinking', if stimulated in a woman who is giving birth, will result in fear and self-consciousness. This leads to the production of adrenaline, a hormone that at this stage of the birthing process inhibits the work of oxytocin, slowing or even stopping the birth. When, in days gone by, we roamed on the plains of Africa, this process worked perfectly. If attacked by a predator, birth could pause while you and your partner ran away. These days an understanding of what slows the birthing process down is important, because you can take action to create the quiet space she needs to birth well.

We know a lot about what encourages abundant oxytocin, just as we understand what can inhibit its flow. The mechanism of release is dependent on a certain mind/body state and is inhibited (in the first stage of the birthing process) by adrenaline in the system. Adrenaline production is predominantly under the control of the neocortex and is stimulated by fear, being watched by others, bright lights and being asked questions that require thinking to answer.

Oxytocin, in this context, is a pacifist and in the face of fear it will run and hide. It is often called the 'shy' hormone! Your lover, as she dances the feminine dance of birth, needs privacy, warmth and deep sensations of comfort and safety. The hormones present at birth are similar to those that make a woman's sexual climax the experience that it is.

Michel Odent, a hugely influential French obstetrician and birth researcher, says that female sexual climax and birth are one event separated by time. A good rule of thumb when thinking about the kind of environment best suited for the birth of your child is to think about the last time your lover enjoyed a deep, rich, noisy – if you were lucky! – orgasm. When you have that thought clearly in mind, remember where you were and take note. Chances are it was private, warm and dimly lit, and as her excitement peaked you were not asking for her opinion on any important subjects.

Oxytocin is stimulated by touch. Massage can encourage more of it to cascade through her body, and yours. Oxytocin is responsible for connections, our sense of loving one another. It also has a role to play in the milk let-down reflex, so it's important as she goes on to feed her baby. (We'll cover this in Chapter 7.)

On the Birthing For Blokes programme that this book is based on we set 'homework' after each session. After the first week each man is asked to offer his partner two massages with oil a week (see Appendix 2) leading up to the birth. He is not to tell her that he has been told to do it, and along with these acts of love he is to think of three other ways that he can express his love for her non-verbally.

When she reaches 37 weeks pregnant the massage should become a sensual one, ideally leading to her experiencing a body-shaking climax. All the time you are restraining yourself from following through on your own excitement: no finishing off on her breasts! This is for her, not you. Your self-sacrifice will send powerful non-verbal messages about your ability to be fully present and focused on her. The discipline required forms part of your training to be present and create a safe space for her later, when the unfolding drama of birth threatens to draw you in and wring you out.

There are at least five benefits of her having regular orgasms at this stage in her pregnancy:

1. She likes it.

2. It causes her uterine muscle to contract, encouraging blood flow to the baby and exercising the muscle.

3. It bathes her brain in the hormone responsible for great birth.

4. It stimulates a sense of togetherness between the two of you.

5. If she is being advised to have the birthing process induced (we will talk about this in a later chapter), it is thought by some that having an orgasm can get things started.

Another exercise that we set for men on the Birthing For Blokes programme involves taking advantage of the way our less-than-conscious mind takes practices that we have repeated over time and causes the mind and body experience created to happen automatically.

---

take action

This week, offer her a massage at least twice.
Use the outline in Appendix 2.

We will talk about this more in a later chapter, but you have probably heard of Dr Pavlov and his dog. The doctor fed his dog each day and at the same time rang a bell. This went on for a number of days until one day Pavlov just rang the bell without offering food. On hearing the bell the dog salivated, thus demonstrating that it is possible to be conditioned to respond in an automatic way when stimulated by repetitive actions.

We ask men to compile a playlist of slow music that he and his lover can dance to. This exercise depends upon his partner finding listening to music relaxing. Once a couple have decided on a playlist they are encouraged to regularly slow dance together throughout the pregnancy.

The discussion so far has probably prompted you to think about the options you and your lover have about the place you choose for her to give birth. The choices open to you are covered in Chapter 4, but what follows is a checklist of action points for you as you create a quiet space for her to give birth in:

- If you are in the hospital you are responsible for making sure that only people truly needed in the birth room are there. Everyone who enters should have knocked and been introduced. If you are at home the power dynamics are different, but the principle is the same.

- Is the room dimly lit? At home you can draw curtains: get blackout material if possible. In hospital if it is daytime you might be able to black out the windows, and you will definitely want to dim the lights.

- Does she have blankets and enough to wear if she needs to keep warm? Is the heating set at a suitable temperature?

- If you are in hospital have you taken something from home that smells familiar and is comforting to her?

- Have you taken the oil in case she wants a massage?

To those of us that have worked in 'maternity' hospitals, it's very clear that our current system of care delivery is not sufficiently sensitive to the ancient processes we have evolved to optimise the survival of the human race. In fact, in hospital we often find the exact opposite of what's needed for great birth to take place: bright lights, strangers, weird smells and lots of waiting around.

Wherever a woman ultimately gives birth, in the early stages of the birthing process she is probably going to do better in a place where she feels comfortable, and where she is used to feeling comfortable: at home. Your main job at this stage – and in one form or another it's been the role of a man for thousands of years – is to keep fear at bay.

what happens for him?

When the woman you love is being taken over by an oxytocin-fuelled trip, you are going to become an adrenaline factory. Why? Because as we have already

take action

Start to find out, secretly if you can, which 'slow' songs your partner likes. You know the ones: in the old days they were the songs played at the end of the disco for couples to smooch to. Compile a slow dance playlist, and in between the massage days, slow dance together.

said, when we were hunter-gathers your birthing lover needed protecting. She still DOES!

Since female human beings have been birthing upright, men have probably been responsible for keeping them safe, both from feelings of fear, as well as the actual threat of attack. Back when predators threatened the life of a newborn, that would have meant a man fighting a wild animal. Now you have a different job: turn the lights down, guard the door and keep her warm.

We have all experienced the impact that a rush of adrenaline has on our minds and bodies: a fast heart rate, breathlessness and, for some, feelings of agitation or impending doom. There can also be an increased sense of focus and heightened levels of energy. It's good to remind yourself that this stress response is instinctive and automatic. You don't have to make it happen, or practise – it works perfectly. When she is about to give birth is the wrong time to be starting to think about how you are going to handle it. This book will give you the tools to keep you grounded when adrenaline wants to drag you off your feet.

2
EVOLUTION, LANGUAGE AND MEANING-MAKING

We are always communicating, even when we think we are not. Our unconscious mind is responsible for much of what we 'say' to others. An understanding that communication happens at different levels will enhance your ability to communicate with everyone in the birth room, but most importantly it will help you support your lover as she gives birth to your child.

Once you have experience in your own life of the interplay between irresistible evolutionary forces and your own unconscious processes as they express themselves in communication, you will be able to extend that gap between stimulus and response, giving you more room to *choose* how you are going to act as the 'birth drama' unfolds. As your understanding deepens, through observation and practice, you will begin to notice how all the others in the birth room are responding to their own unconscious meaning-making patterns, and be able to recognise your own automatic ways of responding.

Paul Ekman, professor emeritus of psychology at the University of California San Francisco School of Medicine, discovered 20 years ago that if a person 'put on their face' one of what he calls the 'universal emotions', they would begin to experience the physiology of that emotion. So smile, and feel happy. This phenomenon is evident in all people regardless of culture or ethnicity.

He concluded that the face is not 'just' a display system that tells others what is happening on the inside (although the fact that the face does act as a display system, along with the rest of your body, opens up many possibilities for really effective rapport-building and deep levels of connection), but that it is also possible to 'self-generate' any emotion by making the movements that constitute the 'end signal' of that emotion on our own face.

Once you understand this, and the principle of multi-level communication, you can introduce safeguards against inappropriate influence, often exerted unknowingly by a medical professional.

Have you ever met someone for the first time, and for reasons you can't put your finger on, you get a sense that you don't like them? You have just experienced a multi-level communication. Your unconscious mind has just done a rapid search of every person you have ever met and decided to give you a signal in consciousness (that feeling) to be careful. Of course at times the signal turns out to be pointing in the wrong direction, and this new 'friend' is nothing like the composite ones you were being warned about. But at other times you'll have had a useful alert to the fact that this person might not be in sympathy with you. (Birth professionals be warned: we are communicating all the time. Our body language, tone and even the way we structure our sentences all influence a pregnant woman's meaning-making.)

There are three forces at work in the 'multi-level' communication that all human beings engage in, which create 'display signals' on our faces, in our bodies and in our words and tones of voices. These are Primeval Forces, Cultural/Social Tribal Forces and Personal Forces – all rooted in deeply unconscious processes, but displayed for all to see, hear and feel.

I do some work in a secure mental health hospital. We had a new 'patient' admitted whom I had never met. As I walked into the lounge, she looked at me intently. She was an older woman of about 70, with staring eyes. She started to smile and chuckle, which is always a little disconcerting. Finally she stopped and laughingly said 'You've just answered a question I've been wondering about all my life'! Bearing in mind that I had never met her before, or said a word yet, I was intrigued. 'What question?' I asked, hesitantly. 'Now I know what Santa does in the summer!' she replied.

I've also recently been to Paris. I'd never been before – it was a birthday treat. Armed only with schoolboy French I found myself in a Parisian 'rugby' bar watching England play France in the Six Nations. The French rugby fans were amazingly warm and friendly, even though my command of French was crap; I had already ordered a pint of fish. Lots of hugging and kissing ensued. It was an amazing evening of friendships forged and victory savoured. At the end of the evening as I got up to leave my new-found friends, I went to the bar to pay my 60 euro bar bill only to find they had already paid it.

Communication is always taking place. That old woman and those French men received a communication from me and I from them. If it had been Paris St Germain playing Leeds United in a football match, I'm guessing I might have got a different kind of 'bar treat'.

primeval forces

Dr Paul Ekman, the psychologist I mentioned earlier, rediscovered seven universal emotional responses that all human beings share, regardless of cultural or social background. I say rediscovered, because Darwin had already expressed a belief that this was so. In the years in between anthropologist Dr Margaret Mead had strongly suggested that Darwin's belief was wrong; her feeling was that all expressions of emotion were culturally prescribed, created as a product of our conditioning.

Dr Ekman lived with a South American 'pre-historic' tribe for three years to test his theory, and what he found has profound implications, not only for our communication with others, but also for our own emotional lives. He discovered that all human beings display, through the muscles on their faces, the seven internal emotional responses, and that these responses are involuntary: they happen in 'split seconds', long before we can control them.

The seven emotions are: anger, fear, sadness, disgust, contempt, surprise and happiness.

Responses to emotion are rooted in the limbic system in our brains (the same part of the brain we spoke about in Chapter 1). It's a much older part of the brain than the neocortex. The limbic system connects us to all other mammals, responding instinctively to outside stimuli. In days gone by these mammalian reactions kept us alive, saving us from being eaten by predators. In our modern lives they propel us out of the way of oncoming cars. As we have said, it's our limbic system that secretes the hormones of love, of which oxytocin is one, which start and keep your lover's birthing process going, and which also conduct the crescendo of our body-shaking orgasms. Let's hear it for the limbic system!

However, the new kid on the block, the neocortex, barely 200,000 years old, wants to get involved in life events like birth and sex. But when the thinking, questioning, meaning-making neocortex tries to help the ancient limbic system out, it screws things up. We've seen this in our discussion of birth and it's the same when it comes to life in general. Our instinctive emotional responses cannot be turned off, and our ability to sense the responses of others is excellent. Without these instincts you wouldn't be here; you are the pinnacle of evolutionary success. You work perfectly.

The neocortex takes our intuitive knowing of what is happening in the people we are communicating with and adds *meaning* to it. When you are speaking to someone, and outside of your conscious awareness you sense they are angry or showing contempt, your meaning-making neocortex says 'They don't like you, they think you are fat, stupid, crap...' This kind of meaning-making creates an internal response in you, which in turn sends a signal back to them... it's a cycle.

This cycle of communication is taking place all the time, and humans spend most of their lives taking other humans' instinctive signals personally. Of course people misunderstand your signals too, and judge you, but their judgement is a completely personal hallucination. When you are being present to your lover as she births, knowing this will give you a deep insight into what is 'controlling' the other human beings (midwife, doctor) in the room.

cultural, social and tribal forces

As if communication was not challenging enough, there is a communication driver which relates to the country, group of people, or tribe we are born into, including, at the micro level, our family. These are conditioned responses that operate as unconscious rules for what's right and wrong. My children and grandchildren are walking in the footsteps I thought I covered up!

Looking back at the Paris story, if I had been in a

football bar and not a rugby bar, I might have been in danger. If I was stupid enough to be wearing an England shirt, different tribal rules could have applied.

We have all heard about distinctive tribal behaviour: promiscuous Inuits getting syphilis, Maasai Mara boys hunting lions to become men and French men wanting to kiss each other. There is always at least one person who is willing to subvert cultural norms, and as they are joined by others a new culture can evolve and grow. Nonetheless, the micro tribal/cultural ways of acting that you and your lover will experience in the birth room are profoundly embedded.

personal forces

Beyond the forces that drive all our communication is a personal force that is creating how you experience life itself: it's a set of ways of 'sensing' the world that you and I have come to mistake as who we actually are.

Every moment we are alive we receive messages, data even, from the 'outside' world. Our data-receiving instruments have been at work for us from as early as eight weeks after our Dads did their orgasmic limbic-system-guided work to fertilise our mothers' eggs.

Our eyes, ears, skin, nose and mouth collect billions of 'bits' of information every millisecond, a dazzling stream of multi-coloured, textured life, rolling in wave after wave. The truth is that it's impossible to for us to sort and store it all. We have to make sense of the vast amount of data coming in, and every human being does this in a unique individual way. What we are left with is an approximation of 'real life', and this is how our personalities develop.

If you ever tried to find your way using a map before the fabulous invention of the sat nav, you will know that it's useful to have a pictorial 'representation' of what the 'territory' should look like. The map approximates the world it represents; the more successfully it does so, the easier it is to find your way.

Your brain does something very similar. It takes the deluge of information being received through your senses, generalises stuff, changes and distorts other bits and deletes whole swathes of it, to create an internal 'map' that you then use to make meaning and sense of what is happening moment to moment.

Have a look at the image above right, which illustrates this process.

Alfred Korbisky, the father of general semantics, pithily reminds us that, 'the map is not the territory', or, put another way, 'the menu is not the meal'. Our tendency as human beings is to confuse our meaning-making with what is *actually happening*. Once we understand that our current experience is internally created and self-generated, we find a new freedom to feel differently about all kinds of life events.

However, just because we *feel* differently about life events, doesn't mean we can *communicate* clearly about

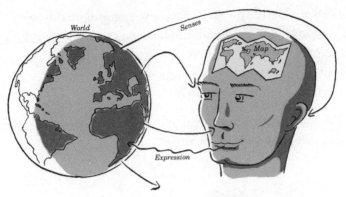

them. The vast majority of human beings spend their relational lives hallucinating that those they speak to totally understand what they are saying with little ambiguity. Do you see in the image above, the 'map' is just a limited, self-created understanding? The thing is, what we communicate is going to be based on that limited understanding.

Have a look at the next image.

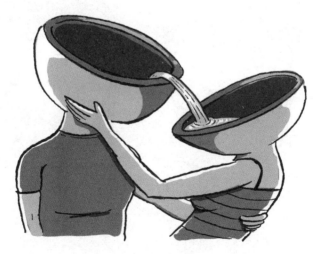

Although this picture gives new meaning to the phrase 'giving head', using this illustration as a mental working model for what is happening as we communicate does little to enhance loving understanding between lovers, friends, and warring countries!

A more accurate, if exaggerated, illustration of what does happen would be this:

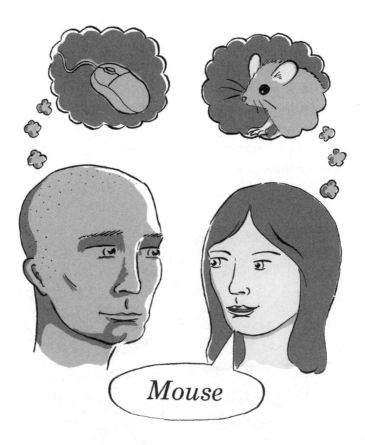

Mouse

As we have already seen, human beings cannot NOT communicate; our bodies send messages constantly. So, work on what you say, how you say it, and on actively listening to what others are trying to say. Remember, their 'map' is not the same as yours.

fostering a loving connection

So why have I spent so much time talking about the importance of communication and how the vast majority of it is happening outside the awareness of those involved? It's because your mission, throughout your lover's pregnancy and subsequent birth, is *to foster a deep connection with your lover.* You can practise ways to help her mind and body to release massive amounts of oxytocin. Being able to manage, proactively, her stress response to life (pregnancy and birth can be an enormously stressful time for a woman, however delighted she may be to be pregnant) is enormously important.

Everything that I discuss is focussed on this one goal: 'connecting' to her. You need to show that you are there, for her and with her, to listen to her without

---

take action

This week take time to notice what's *not* being done around the house. *Do at least one thing.* Don't tell her you are going to do it, and don't tell her when you've done it. Don't look for praise for doing it.

---

interruption, to put your phone down, to respond to things around your home that need doing without being asked, to watch movies together, to massage her, to *never* appear tired or bored when she is expressing concerns about her pregnancy, to never rush to read up on things and 'fix' her. You can start by picking an area in your own life that you have been *saying* you are going to change. Make it a personal thing that she knows about, but don't say anything to her, just start taking some action to change. She will notice and oxytocin will rise in her. It's a great place to start fulfilling your connection mission.

I hope that reading this chapter has given you insights into your lover's unique ways of making meaning in the world. You know her, you love her, she is about to mother your child. Taking this communication stuff and learning more deeply about how to connect to her is not going to be easy! And, as we are going to see later, there will be more than one woman in the birth room – most midwives don't have beards, right?

Like driving a car, the skills for strategically being able to generate this kind of connection with others take time to learn. At first you will have to be conscious of what you are looking for. Later you will be surprised that you are able to observe many things at once without having to concentrate on them at all.

This chapter has been an introduction to multi-level communication (see the bibliography for more reading) and we don't have space to go into endless detail about reading distinctive body postures, breathing patterns and eye movements that can give you enough information to truly understand how the person you are connecting with is making meaning in their world. For now, try to notice the describing words others use, then offer them words back from the same family of sensory descriptive words. What do I mean? Here is an example. She says 'I can't *see* the way forward with this pregnancy, it's not *clear* to me how it's going to work out, I just can't *picture* giving birth'. Which of her five senses is she favouring? Yep, 'seeing'. When you respond to her, use similar words. She is much more likely to feel that you've understood her. Try it out, and 'see', 'hear' and 'feel' the difference. Below and on the next page are lists of the words for each sense to look out for. She will use words from all five senses, but a preference will stand out.

meaning-making words

Visual words: hazy, obscure, dim, film, opacity, perspective, cloudiness, focus, picture, envision, vision, viewpoint, view, look, gaze, illuminate, glimpse, illustrate, perceive, watch, scan, survey, visible, glance, glare, stare, show, pretty, clear, glow

Auditory words: hear, listen, talk, harmony, noisy, call, loud, shout, told, dissonance, resounding, lend an ear, amplify, cadence, chatter, whine, moan, hiss, groan, voice, acoustics, sounds like, cry, silence, tune, tone, scream   *...continues*

Kinesthetic words: feel, warm, touch, handle, grasp, soft, tight, smooth, rough, firm, pressure, tense, concrete, hurt, roughly, clumsy, relaxed, swell, tremble, shiver, shake, penetrate, absorb, grope, stir, agitated, cutting, flush, itch, creeps

Gustatory/olfactory words: taste, flavour, savour, relish, tangy, palatable, odour, aftertaste, smell, scent, whiff, pungent, stink, reek, a nose for, leave a bad taste.

Another communication hack involves observing how the person you are connecting with is 'holding' their body. 'Body language' would be a shorthand way of saying this, but the trouble is that the whole idea of body language and meaning has been over-used and is probably crap. You know the type of thing: she's crossing her arms, therefore she is 'closed'. Bollocks, she could be cold, hiding a stain on her uniform, giving herself a cleavage... who knows? All you can know for sure is that when she is crossing her arms, one arm is crossed over the other! (Deep, eh?)

Human beings are remarkably consistent. Our thoughts and feelings will always leak out through BMW: our Bodies (postures) Music (tone of voice) and our Words. What we see on the outside is the fruit of an internal process. When you offer someone a mirror image of themselves on the outside, in most circumstances the connection between you is strengthened.

These communication techniques take practice. Don't worry, you've got time – up to nine months if your lover is already pregnant, longer if you're reading this before conceiving a child.

From now on, when you are at work, out shopping, talking to friends, and being with your lover, start to watch and listen closely. Remember BMW. People are *always* telling you what type of language they prefer to receive information in. Listen to their words. When you start to talk their language, they will respond.

---

take action

When you are talking to her this week, take the time to hear which one of her senses she seems to prefer and begin to offer her those words back in conversation. Also, notice her body posture, the angle of her head tilt, whether her legs are crossed. Slowly begin to mirror her posture. Don't tell her what you're doing, but notice how she responds to you. For a contrasting experience, deliberately do the opposite and notice what happens. Don't tell her about your experiments, but see what happens to the connection between you each time. You've got to be careful; subtle even. If the person gets any sense that you are mimicking them, connection will be broken. Start by mirroring half body positions. What are they doing with their arms and upper body? Can you reflect that? What happens when you do?

3

THE MASCULINE AND FEMININE DANCE OF BIRTH

Based on his experience of men entering the birth room and his understanding of the evolutionary biological adaptations of birthing women, Dr Michel Odent says that men should stay out of the way when women give birth. I get where he is coming from. One of the most important decisions you will ever make is whether you want to be in the birth room when she gives birth or not, though let's be honest: these days it's expected of you. However, lying to yourself and others when you are really feeling like you would prefer to be outside will backfire big time.

Given what we've said about the multi-level nature of communication, you can be sure that if you don't want to be there she will know, subconsciously or consciously. You can't hide fear, discomfort and anxiety, no matter how hard you try, and because she knows you so well, she can smell it. If, in the midst of the birthing process, she senses your discomfort, it will inhibit the process of her losing herself in the flood of oxytocin, and she will worry about your wellbeing. If she doesn't mother you already she will start doing it then, at a time when her baby needs all of her. What she needs from you when she is giving birth is not much different from what she wants on a day-to-day basis: she wants a sense of connection, and this felt sense of connection stimulates a flood of oxytocin.

Being orgasmic is a fabulous source of oxytocin. (Pornography has a lot to answer for: women should get more orgasms than they do. It should not surprise us that a masculine-influenced birthing system is goal-orientated, as when it comes to sex most men think that way too.) If she is lucky enough to climax when you have sex, great, but don't suggest sex when she is feeling stressed. She is likely to hurt you! What she needs is a reservoir of oxytocin to even feel like getting it on with you in the first place. You doing the washing up, putting out the rubbish and listening to her without trying to 'fix' the problem she is sharing creates an environment in which her oxytocin levels can rise.

As we have already said, female orgasm and birth can be viewed as one event separated by time. When she is birthing she wants you there, doing only the things that will enhance the felt sense of connection between you. She is your lover, you are the man she has chosen over others to spend her life with, and to start or grow a family with. During birth the sense of connection she has with you, along with the process of birth itself, will cause her oxytocin levels to soar.

As men we should constantly be asking 'Will what I am saying or doing have an impact on her oxytocin levels? Will my actions and words create a connection?' Don't get me wrong, you're not responsible for her biochemistry. Every man and woman in the world has the same set of hormones, but how these interact and work in men and women is different. I'm not wanting to stereotype, but it's worth noting that the stereotypes originated as a result of this gender-specific hormonal balance resulting in certain types of behaviour.

Dr Odent acknowledges that in his experience men went from being 'present at birth, to participating in the birth'. He suggests that early in his experience of men being present in the birth room births seemed to go well, and he explains why he thinks women started to want their partners to be present. He outlines key changes in how birth became industrialised, and centred in big maternity hospitals, at the same time as a sociological downsizing of the extended family occurred. Birth moved from being a family-centred activity that happened at home, to being an impersonal process, measured by men, that was managed in a large factory (hospital). Of course women wanted someone in the room that they felt close to, and, to start with, having the father present worked: his presence was what she needed as a kind of antidote to the birth machinery around her. But then something changed: men began to get involved in the nitty-gritty of the birth process.

Men, like their largely male obstetrician brothers,

began to think of pregnancy and birth as a problem needing a fix. They started to lose themselves in obstetric detail, and being men they could empathise with the medical model on show. This objectification of childbirth put up a wall between men and women and their important connection was lost. The knowledge of what could go wrong (which is emphasised in a medical model) led to fear-induced activity. This does not foster deep connection, because she senses the fear. Some neurophysiologists claim that because a woman has more connections between the two hemispheres of the brain (corpus callosum), this leads to her being able to process many more subjects at once, while a man, with his limited connection points, seeks to focus on one issue in order to settle his sense of overload. This physical phenomenon may be an explanation for the idea that men can't multi-task and women can, as has long been believed in popular culture.

As a woman watches and listens to how her lover is responding as the dance of the birthing process begins to unfold, consciously and unconsciously, if she has a man in the room who needs her, her deeply embedded maternal instincts are evoked in his interest. She is shaken out of the deep trance needed for oxytocin release, and, as Odent reports, the birthing process is slowed. However, Dr Odent has observed that often, when the man leaves the room for some reason, the woman promptly finds her primeval self again and the birthing process proceeds very quickly to the birth of the baby.

As men we can be forgiven for making this mistake. But we need to recognise how birth has, to some extent, been hijacked by men. The 'system' of birth has been designed by men. We recognise, and are reassured by, the pattern of problem solving. It's deeply unconscious and written into our genetic coding. It's no wonder we are afraid of birth: people we respect, and masculine-orientated information that we trust, have been telling us it's dangerous for years. We can be forgiven for not knowing better until now. But now we know what it takes to truly support a woman, we have no excuse for not acknowledging our responsibilities as lover and father-to-be.

How do you prepare to give this kind of presence to her as she gives birth? The same way you keep your

---

doulas

What if she needs or wants support from another woman? What if you need help to support your lover? A doula might be the answer

In her book *Why Doulas Matter* (Pinter & Martin, 2015) Maddie McMahon explains how dads and doulas can be a 'dream team':

When I work with a couple, I try hard to get across the message that, in fact, the partner has a crucial part to play. His feelings about his role, and what she wants and needs from him, are important to share. If they are a loving couple, the oxytocin they can produce together, as they gaze into each other's eyes, kiss, cuddle and touch, is more powerful

---

than any artificial hormone drip. He can be home, safety, privacy, labour progression, lover, advocate and protector all rolled into one. But he doesn't have to always be by her side to give her exactly what she needs.

...For a woman, having her significant other there with her on this amazing day can be incredible. The love and connection that put the baby in there, can really help to get the baby out. But equally, I've known fathers who do not wish to be there, or at least not in an active role. I've met women who love their partner dearly, but laugh at the idea of having him present, or know that it will be beyond his capabilities to support her in the way she needs. There is no judgement in that knowledge; why should there be? You may encounter people who have strong opinions about men in the birthing room. I think it's time we moved away from old-fashioned notions of gender. Instead we should ask, 'Will this person bring oxytocin or adrenaline into the room?' and 'What do the parents want?'

During my years of doulaing I've met many fathers. Sometimes it's the father who makes the initial call. The myth that doulas are only there for the mother and can even have a negative effect on the ability of the father to support his partner persists. But it isn't what I see.

Take the father who remembered trying to support his wife first time round in the hospital. He had no idea how best to comfort and support her, and they had been left alone for long periods of time in the busy delivery unit. No one offered him drinks or snacks and he didn't feel he could leave his wife. Frankly, he'd been terrified and, after a long labour and birth, was faint with hunger and dehydration. This time, he wanted a help-mate and companion. I tended to them both when she went into labour. I fed and watered them, fetched and carried, made the tea, showed him how to massage her back, to dance with her during the *contractions, to love and care for her through each surge until the baby made his entrance.*

...Of course, it's often the woman who wants the doula. It's not uncommon for the father to not really understand why. Usually they just want their partner to be happy and comfortable, so will happily welcome the doula into the birth space. It's my job to make sure his fears and anxieties are addressed and that he feels supported too.

It can sometimes be a challenge for a father to understand his wife's preferences and choices. Why would she dream of a normal birth after the frightening labour and emergency c-section last time? Why would she risk planning to stay at home to have the baby? Why does she want to invite this strange woman to share our private journey? Isn't formula-feeding a simpler, more controlled and measurable way to feed the baby, that will enable him to help her?

Inviting a doula to participate in these discussions can help facilitate effective communication, and allow mutual understanding to grow and concerns to be put into context. A doula may provide the father with evidence-based reading material, or suggest a health professional to talk to so that he understands the risks and benefits of his partner's choices. The result is a birth 'dream team' – two sets of hands to support her, two loving companions to hold her birth space and have faith in her ability to birth this baby beautifully.

If you've read this and think a doula might be for you, talk to your partner about it. You can find out about hiring a doula on the Doula UK website. Cost isn't necessarily a barrier – if you're strapped for cash there are schemes that aim to make doula support accessible to everyone.

relationship with her rocking and rolling on a day-to-day basis. If you are not having sex very often and wanking is losing its appeal, stimulating her oxytocin levels will be the biggest gift you can give yourself and her. Take every opportunity to cement your loving connection with her. Remember that she is living in a world that is testosterone-saturated. Testosterone is an antagonist to oxytocin and increases her stress. After a day at work, the activities that would ordinarily boast her oxytocin levels, like cooking, eating and keeping her home environment how she likes it, become just more 'things to do'. It needs to be said again at this point that gender stereotypes are crap, but an understanding of the way our endocrine (hormonal) system runs the show can lead to enlightened behaviour in both men and women. Equality is not at issue here. After 70 million years of evolutionary development, you can bet that biochemical forces are shaping our actions at an instinctive level. Because of our neocortex we imagine ourselves to be superior animals, so we tell ourselves stories about our behaviour and the reasons behind it, when the truth is that it is largely down to involuntary processes.

Back to our goal: for her to experience our 'masculine presence' and a felt sense of safety and connection. This will enable the 'feminine' to express herself with abandon, to surrender to the pulsations of life as the baby is born. The unfolding narrative will be unhindered by fear.

Today male partners are present at 95 per cent of all births. What men need is an understanding of how they can use their masculine presence in such a way that the women they love do not feel observed. Masculine presence can act like a 'cloak', covering her so that the freedom of darkness can be unleashed.

Masculine and feminine 'energy' (for want of a better word; my girlfriend calls me a 'spiritual wanker' when I use words like 'energy', 'awareness' and 'grounded' – I say it's difficult finding words that fit the experience I'm attempting to communicate) are not only physical body issues; they are rooted in a physiological, endocrine system-driven hormonal dance that profoundly influences our human relationships.

Being able as men to create an environment where she feels safe and connected to others – and us – relies in part on the physical environment, but our focussed attention on her, which encourages oxytocin, is even more important.

The behaviours that have been characterised as 'masculine' and 'feminine' operate as a directional force, influencing how life is being experienced from moment to moment. We see life through our neuro-physiological filters.

There are obvious differences in how these hormonal forces express themselves. Dr John Grey popularised this understanding in his book *Men are from Mars, Women are from Venus*. He has since updated his work in *When Mars and Venus Collide*, adding this foundational physiological understanding of our endocrine systems.

Men and women respond very differently to stress, and this is borne out by current research. When a woman gets stressed she produces higher levels of testosterone, which stops our old friend oxytocin from doing its work, not just during birth, but in all aspects of life.

It seems that the world has changed for women, and reports of stress-related illness are increasing. A woman needs to be bathed in oxytocin in order to relax and refill her energy banks for another day. For men it's different: when testosterone increases in us, our stress levels begin to *lower*. The masculine tendency to engage in adrenaline-fuelled sports and pastimes to relax makes sense in this context. In fact, any testosterone-stimulating activity will enable us to unwind. By age 50 the levels of testosterone in our bodies have halved, and some studies suggest that there is a direct link between dropping testosterone levels and an increase in depression in men. When we experience this kind of testosterone reduction, not only do we have a hard time getting hard, we often feel aimless and overly tired. Testosterone in our system inhibits the working of oestrogen, and when testosterone falls, oestrogen increases, which in turn affects our zest for life.

All this seems very obvious when someone points it out, but until they do we are often stuck using approaches that don't work to communicate with people we meet.

A person with a masculine essence, for example, will respond better to challenge than to praise. Someone rich in female energy will flourish when praised and offered appreciation. There are many situations in which knowing this can make communicating your message much easier and more effective. In general, attempting to motivate your lover through challenge is likely to cause her to turn off and reject your offering.

So what's a man to do? How can you prepare for the birthing process in such a way that she will get a rich sense of you being there for her, like a protective superhero, generating an invisible forcefield encompassing all three of you, at this amazingly exciting but potentially fight or flight-generating time?

One answer is to care for yourself first. Anything that has a tendency to reduce your testosterone levels will, over time, increase your stress levels. I know you've heard all this before, but when I heard it in the context of how my mind and body works, and has done for millions of years, it changed my perspective and made making the needed changes easier.

Think about your sleep patterns. How much sleep are you getting each night? What would you say is the quality of that sleep? If you know you are getting crap sleep and not enough of it, do something about it. Black the room out, wear a mask to sleep in, get into a routine. Go to bed at the same time and get up at the same time. Good sleep will help to restore testosterone levels.

Do some research around food and testosterone levels (and see the bibliography for more reading). Bear in mind that some foods increase oestrogen levels in men, and higher oestrogen levels are antagonistic to testosterone. Milk is one example. On the other hand, some foods boost testosterone levels: try eggs, grapes, avocados, pomegranates, garlic, venison and cabbage.

If you are not already exercising, start. Twenty minutes a day is a good starting point. Research suggests that although slow cardiovascular exercise like brisk walking is always a good thing, the kind of exercise that boosts testosterone is short bursts of high-intensity activity, like skipping, circuit training or sprinting (you may need a medical check before embarking on a new high-intensity activity). If you're anything like me, you might be sighing inside at this point and thinking, 'Fuck, I've tried this kind of approach to my health before and I've failed.' You haven't done this before. It's likely that this is the first time you have realised that your body has been in development for millions of years and that it will function best when you treat it and feed it in a certain way. Let this knowledge transform your levels of enthusiasm and motivation, and take action today. Hell, if you can't do it because your lover and child need you to, at least look forward to the rock-hard erections, and do the necessary research!

If your waist is over 35 inches (mine is at the moment, but since really getting into this stuff I have lost weight, which has boosted my energy and zest for life no end), the fat in your stomach is producing oestrogen, and we now know what that means. Lowered testosterone. So if you need too, start to lose weight.

The research is mixed about whether smoking lowers testosterone levels. No one knows for sure. But if she doesn't smoke and you do, stopping will send an amazing message and increase her oxytocin levels. She'll get the message 'He cares for me and he is concerned for the health of our baby' and you'll increase your own sense of wellbeing. Focussing on overcoming the habit will raise your testosterone levels for sure, and probably increase your and your baby's life expectancy. Just do it. There is support available from the NHS, and vaping (e-cigarettes) is now the fastest-growing method for stopping smoking in the UK. The online vaping community is a source of great advice.

Vaping probably reduces the harm in smoking by 95 per cent, and with the right concentration of nicotine you still get the same buzz, smell good and get to live longer. And in the mind of your lover, you'll be a god-like figure with iron will power!

I hate to mention alcohol, but you already know the truth. If you're drinking heavily, there are reasons for that. You're self-medicating for the stresses in your life and work. Alcohol itself also reduces testosterone levels. If you're drinking for the feeling of calm after a busy day, consider drinking smarter: have a small whisky instead of four cans of lager. Try using the buzz-inducing effects of short bursts of intense exercise to de-stress instead. Although talking to our men friends doesn't give us the same stress-relieving effects that women get from talking to their female friends, having a couple of mates who will offer us a challenge in these areas will raise our testosterone levels. So speak to a friend, make yourself accountable for what you say you want to do and ask him to support you. Actually no, tell him to kick your butt if you get off track.

Thinking about 'accountability', review your work habits with a couple of mates. When we are in a stress-filled 'rut' it's often difficult to see and think our own way out of it. Tell them straight how much you are working, talk about any money worries you have, set measurable goals and get your mates to coach you through taking action. Words are *very* cheap; actions are what truly count. In fact, if you've read this and feel an intense sense of motivation to take action, put the book down, pick up your phone and arrange to meet a mate to talk through this stuff you just read.

Don't tell your partner what you are going to do. She has almost certainly heard it all before and seen you wimping out on taking action. As you start to make changes, she will notice. As you become the man that can offer her and your growing family the security she feels she needs, her oxytocin levels will increase and her stress will reduce. It's the very best preparation for birth and becoming parents.

You can also prepare yourself mentally. I don't want to get too 'New Age' on you, but there is some evidence that being able to settle your mind, or at least to become still enough to notice the incessant internal chatter (you might call it thinking), that trundles along all the time just below awareness, can have positive benefits.

Your lover will not be the only woman in the birth room. Midwives, medics and maternity support workers will connect with you and your lover more effectively if their oxytocin levels are topped up too. What can you do to increase oxytocin levels in the room as a whole? (NB: I am *not* suggesting that you offer to massage the midwife!)

Talk about this stuff with your partner, and think through ways you could begin to make a connection with the women caring for her. Ideally you would know your midwife already, but to be honest in the NHS at the moment it is unlikely, and often the midwife will be unknown to you both. You could put together a box as a gift for her, and pack some treats for her to eat. Offer her words of appreciation often, and remember the context in which she is caring for you. She will be working hard, so her testosterone levels are sure to be raised. Think again about multi-level communication: she will be sending you unconscious signals, giving you clues as to how she is making her own internal map of 'reality'. We discussed those signals earlier, and as part of your preparation you will have practised reading them, so now you are in a position to offer her an experience of deep connection with you both.

take action

Discuss with your lover the idea of buying small gifts to give to the midwives (you might have more than one – even several – depending on shift patterns). Sweets, hand cream, drinks and small, inexpensive gifts might be suitable. Ask your partner's opinion, and between you agree to buy these things and have them ready before the birth process starts.

I want you to be focussed on your job in the room. Your goal, your mission, your task in the room is to offer your lover yourself, seeking always to connect deeply. As we have said, when she truly 'feels' this, her oxytocin levels will rise.

So far we have been exploring how a man can be as prepared as possible for imminent fatherhood, and how you can ready yourself through actions that you begin to take today which will give you the edge when the birthing process starts. If you've already begun to take action, I expect you have noticed the difference in the levels of intimacy and connection you and your lover are experiencing. The sooner you begin to prepare, and the more you do, the better it will be for you both when the birth process gets under way and her body begins to do its thing. This type of connection-building action produces a relationship between the two of you that will be an amazingly secure foundation for your new family.

In the next chapter you are going to sit in on a group session with men preparing for birth. Some of the themes have already been discussed, so you may hear things you already know, restated in different ways and expanded in response to real questions that men are asking. You will also see the answers to specific questions men raise about pregnancy and birth itself. A men's group session can be really helpful, because your main mission, as I've said already, is to respond to the questions *she* is asking. When she has finished thinking things through, you'll have your own questions – you're a man, right? – and talking those through with other men, as well as with her (when she's ready) can help you to feel well prepared for what's ahead.

4
A CONVERSATION WITH MEN

This group session is a starting point for discussions you and your lover might have about her experience of birth and her interaction with the various structures of birth. A word of caution, though: resist the temptation to become an 'expert' on birth. It's better to engage with all the birthing education material from a different perspective, asking: 'How can I use this new knowledge to build a sense of human beings connecting when I'm in the birth room?' Most men, when presented with a new area to master, have a tendency to want to be an expert, to know stuff, to be able to argue for what's right, to correct and challenge: and this is great in different contexts. It's probably why you are good at your job, snowboarding or making stuff, but when your child is being born getting lost in this will not help. Any sense of challenge will quickly build a wall between you and the midwife, and your partner will sense it and feel unsettled.

Use your imagination as you read the discussion: ask yourself, 'What more do I need to know about that? How can I take action in this area?' When you don't

---

take action

When talking to your lover about her pregnancy, listen for anything she says relating to worries or fears about the birth. If she raises questions about stuff you don't know about, find out about it, but not with the goal of just sharing your knowledge. Remember that being *connected* to her is your primary goal. Show her that you are deeply interested; share an opinion – but give her time to make up her own mind and consider her own response to the information. Her conclusions will probably be richer than yours, and by not rushing her or trying to 'fix it' you will deepen your connection with her.

---

understand something, or want to know more about it, write down your question or put it in your phone. My email address is at the back of the book, or you can message me on Twitter. Ask. Reading alone never transformed anyone: it's only as you *act* that things and circumstances change.

The names used here are not real, but the men and their questions are. Let's get started.

Daryce: I've been sent here by my girlfriend. I'm not really sure what the group is all about. [Knowing glances round the group, this is very common. Women often send men to me. What she wants is for you to connect and get involved.]

Mark: Thanks for being so straightforward! This group offers you an opportunity to prepare as thoroughly as possible for the challenging job of supporting your lover as she gives birth to your baby.

It's all really about preparing you to be 'present' with her when she gives birth. And by present I'm not talking just about proximity, I'm talking about full-on focussed *presence*. If you put laser-like attention on connecting with her during the birth process, it has the incredible effect of increasing the levels of the hormones she has evolved to make birth work perfectly.

As you learn the skills and ways of understanding necessary to master this 'way of being' with her, it will seem like you have a superpower: you can generate a kind of protective bubble encompassing you and her. You being present creates 'space', or a 'container', for all that's going to happen.

It sounds a little like New Age bullshit, I know – but I'm telling you, having been around birthing couples since 1994, when a man can do this for his family, magic happens in the room. A woman can be surrounded by people but feel as though she's alone with the man she loves. This intimacy allows her to respond to the birth process naturally, like mammals have been doing for millions of years.

Joe: That sounds good, but I've got loads of questions. How will I know labour has started? When do I call the midwife? She keeps talking about 'the show' and I don't know what she's on about!

Mark: Good questions, Joe, and we'll get on to some of them later. I'm going to give you a list of books, YouTube clips and so on that you can use for research if you want to, but in my experience the biggest challenge for us men is that we easily get drawn into the 'drama' of birth. We've evolved a hormonal response that works brilliantly most of the time: for us, a drama poses a challenge to be solved, or something broken to fix. That's often fine, but not for birth!

If our attention is on 'fixing' what's happening in the process of birth, we will neglect the most important mission we have while she is giving birth: maintaining a connection with her.

There's information that you need to know, for sure; but if you get caught up with 'information' when she's actually giving birth you will lose touch with what it means to be truly *with* her.

You can't wait to develop the kind of connection we're talking about; you need to nurture it right through pregnancy. Having conversations with her about her worries about pregnancy and birth is an important way for you to build this kind of connection.

Ben: I find it very hard to listen to her talking about her worries. Often she'll be undecided about something, and I'm just thinking, 'For God's sake, it's obvious what we need to do!'

Mark: We've all been there mate! I hope you just thought it and didn't say it... There have been some recent neurological studies that suggest that women have more connections between the two hemispheres of the brain, perhaps as many as eight times more. This sheds light on why women are able to make so many connections, to talk around a subject, considering it from different perspectives. Men, with fewer connections, tend to hone in on the specifics. We see very quickly what 'we think' is needed to fix the 'problem'.

If we are going to start creating the kind of intimacy needed for her to trust us when things are becoming acute later on, we need to bite our tongue, listen until she is finished and not offer a fix until prompted.

I heard Dr John Grey say once that in the US there are more therapists than there are doctors and nurses put together. Counselling is a billion-dollar industry and 70 per cent of that money is spent by women. British women are not that different! Women will *pay* to be listened to. So start to do it.

Noah: This is my second child, and I'm here because when Jack was born I felt largely disenfranchised when I was in the delivery room. Even before that I felt that I was tolerated at best.

Mark: Much of the research work done in this area sadly confirms what you experienced. Men often report the feelings that you describe. If they didn't feel left out of the birth education process, they expressed frustration at feeling like an afterthought throughout the pregnancy and like an intrusive presence in the birth room itself.

If we are not prepared for this type of experience, as

men we are likely to want to attack the people who we perceive are the source of the problem. This is an instinctive evolved response, which is responsible for the four F's: fight, flight, freeze and 'reproduction'. Once the instinct is aroused it's a difficult 'wild animal' to get back in its box. If it didn't work so well, our ancestors would have died out long ago. To harness the beast we must prepare.

From an evolutionary point of view, if you look at the biological, hormonal adaptations humans have made, the part of the brain responsible for a woman's birthing well is the limbic system; a part of the brain that's a lot older than the neocortex, which is your 'thinking' brain.

The limbic system is quite a primitive part of the brain; it's the mammalian part of the brain. If she can dial down her neocortex, she can unlock that mammalian power to birth instinctively.

Luca: You mean she's in a natural animal state?

Mark: Exactly. Let's be honest, if a man needs anything, he needs confidence in the way the birthing process has worked for millions of years, and an understanding of how it works.

In most sessions I start off by saying, 'You are living proof that the birthing process works perfectly, because you're here. If it didn't work perfectly, you wouldn't be here; it's as simple as that.'

Evolutionary biologists tell us that evolutionary adaptation is incredibly slow and takes many generations. Biologically speaking you are a Stone Age man living in the fast lane, and she's a Stone Age woman living in the fast lane. The way her body responds intuitively to birth is actually the same as it has been for thousands of years.

Once we understand that, and we understand what it takes for her to be able to dip down into that state of consciousness, to enter the limbic system, then what's required when it comes to birth becomes very clear.

We live in a society in which doctors try to convince us that we need them in order to give birth. What we've seen over the years is a medicalisation of the birthing process, and if we want to get a little bit political it's driven predominantly by the male gender, or 'male energy' if you like. So we now have a situation where men in particular are highly aware of what they perceive to be the risks when it comes to birth.

Hey, we get that, right? We know how they feel. When there appears to be a problem, it's got to be fixed, and we can see clearly what needs to be done! If you work in any kind of business, you've probably heard phrases like, 'What gets measured, gets done', or Henry Ford's famous quote 'Obstacles are those frightful things you see when you take your eyes off the goal'. They're great sayings, but valuable in a different context.

Males are goal-fixated. Focussing on an objective has

a massive impact on our testosterone levels. Speak to any depressed man and you'll notice straight away that his sense of purpose has been lost. He is lethargic, directionless and deeply unhappy, and if he were to have blood tests done, we'd find low testosterone levels.

Historically men have attempted to influence the birthing process (their intentions have been good, in the main). If you spend time observing birth you can easily see the results. Men invented 'stages of labour', (more on this later), positions for women to get in to make it easier to use their tools (for example, needing the woman to have her legs in stirrups so the doctor can use forceps). Gadgets and men have tended to go together when it comes to birth.

Don't get me wrong, doctors have their place, and in limited circumstances the work they do saves lives. They make the small number of pregnancies where the ancient birthing physiology has been disrupted by genetic mutation or western lifestyle safer.

But back to your question: the short answer is YES!

Luca: You've got me going now. When you talk about birth being politicised, is it overtly political or is it the politics of the masculine and the feminine?

Mark: Well I think it's true to say that a masculine 'endocrine balance' and a feminine one are not necessarily just binary (digital... what I mean is, not just 'on' or 'off', or one or the other), there is a continuum of how individual people experience their own biochemistry. Dr Grey points to studies that suggest that 90 per cent of men and women experience this endocrine mix of hormones in predictable ways when it comes to resulting behaviours; in his book *When Mars and Venus Collide* he suggests that stereotyping probably results from the consistency of this evolved mechanism, based on the distribution of skills needed to keep us all alive when we were hunter-gatherers.

I read an article in the *Guardian* that suggested that an anthropologist, while exploring the potential for this kind of message to be used in a patriarchal way to oppress women, observed that societies that haven't changed much since our hunter-gatherer days operate on very egalitarian principles. Cooperation was probably a necessity before we started growing food. My left-wing socialist friends would argue that 'profit' in our economy has led to the ongoing exploitation of women.

Given that we all have these hormones working in different ways in our bodies, creating an array of behaviours, we still cannot help but notice that people have a kind of dominant expression, or direction to their behavior. Being a little reductionist, I mean that they have either a masculine essence or a feminine essence.

I have female friends that have a predominantly masculine essence, and I have male friends that have a feminine essence. When it comes to birth, obviously it's the quintessential expression of the feminine.

Now what I would say is that over the years – in the last 30–40 years – in terms of the birth environment a masculine expression, if you like, has taken control. So for example we have what doctors call stages of labour: latent phase, first stage, second stage, third stage. We made up these measurement points, forgot that *we made them up* and now believe them like they're the law.

Aiden: Almost like time itself?

Mark: Say more Aiden, what do you mean like time itself?

Aiden: I was reading somewhere about all how all 'measurements' of any kind, including 'time', have been made up: miles, inches, metres and shit. The physical world is just there, the earth goes round the sun – it was mankind that made up the units to measure what was there already.

Mark: Ah, I get it. Yes, like time, inches and metres, talking about 'stages of labour' is an illusion that's useful, but not if we're bound by it. I do want you to understand what is meant by 'stages of labour', about the latent phase, the first stage, the second stage and the third stage, and we're going to talk about that as the session goes on.

But the first thing to understand is that all of that stuff is manufactured: it's created *ex nihilo*, if you like, out of nothing, and then we are taught to believe it implicitly, like it's the truth.

The male way of fixing stuff is to count and quantify. I don't think there's any denying that.

James: Can you say that again? It's the male tendency to measure?

Mark: Males have a tendency to want to measure, to quantify and to judge distance. I would say that it flows from our male hormonal mix, and particularly form testosterone, which is such an important hormone for men. Measuring, bringing order and being spatially aware are testosterone-stimulated actions. In contrast hormones such as oxytocin and oestrogen are predominantly associated with feminine strength and stress relief. These hormones are stimulated by a sense of narrative, story and deep connection.

You know, it's a good starting point to think of your joint experience of your unique pregnancy and coming birth as a story. Inside that story, that metaphor, a deep connection can begin to be forged as soon as you get home. Storytelling and connection are home turf for these incredibly important female hormones. Given that each story is unique and special, at times both partners may clash with a system that treats everybody the same. Get prepared, oh warrior man!

I'm in danger of going on too long about this hobby horse of mine! Rather than the 'categorising' that goes on at the moment, the whole system that has been built around birth needs a complete overhaul. Women should be right at the centre of that transformation. We will

take action

Writing your birth story, in the way you imagine you would like it to unfold, can be a rewarding experience that will give you and your partner insight into what matters to you about the birth. If you're arty, you could draw instead. You'll hear a lot about 'birth plans' but thinking of birth as an unfolding narrative rather than an event you can plan can be a more helpful way of looking at it. (Later we'll discuss birth preferences – it is helpful to be aware of the choices that are available.)

be talking about the best place to have your baby later, but if you choose home you really become the narrators of the birth story you want to tell.

Chris: Home?! Fuck, you're scaring me now! She's already mentioned it and I reacted quite harshly, I'm afraid. I don't want to put my baby at risk. Surely hospital must be safer than my back room?

Mark: I get where you're coming from, Chris. It's interesting because there's actually been some really good, recent research into this that might change your thinking. When I was born home birth was normal and hospital birth was considered unusual. It was reserved for a small number of complicated pregnancies. Since a government paper called the Peel Report was published in 1971, most births have taken place in hospital. The

Birthplace Study 2011, conducted by the National Perinatal Epidemiology Unit in Oxford (NPEU), looked again at the question of where to give birth. Below I'm going to give you a summary of the findings, which were published in 2014; you can find more detail about them, information I've quoted directly from the study, in the box on pages 83-84.

Giving birth is generally safe; there are only 4.3 negative birth events per 1,000 births.

If you are having your first baby together, choosing to give birth in a midwife-led unit is as safe as giving birth in a doctor-managed hospital.

Giving birth in a doctor-managed hospital leads to more chance of your partner having a caesarean section (operation) and other unnecessary medical interventions during the birthing process.

Your partner has more chance of having a 'normal birth' in a midwife-led unit.

If you are planning your first baby at home there is a 9.3 in 1,000 chance of a negative birth event happening in the birthing process, as compared to a 5.3 in 1,000 rate in a doctor-managed hospital. 45% of women need to transfer to hospital in the midst of the birthing process.

As we've already discussed, given the impact that a *quiet place* has on birth unfolding well, planning for a birth in a midwifery unit might seem the best option.

But you may not want to rule out a home birth given

the study's findings. The 45% transfer rate refers to moving into hospital and not to actual negative birth events. Reasons for making a move into hospital are varied and include the birthing process taking a long time, and the desire for more pain relief (both of which are more common for first-time mothers).

The Birthplace Study looks at women with 'low risk' pregnancies. If your partner has any medical problems that are affecting her pregnancy, getting specialist advice is the place to start as you seek to make up your minds about where to give birth.

I hope that reading this has begun to open up your thinking in a number of ways, stimulating many questions about your joint choice regarding where you want your baby to be born, and a sense of growing peace that you have the power to make these decisions. The way that medics, and to some extent midwives, are trained tends to focus them on the potential *risks,* rather than what we know about the environment that is most likely to lead to an uncomplicated birth.

I think it bears highlighting that this study acknowledges that birth at home can not only be *as safe* as in a doctor-managed hospital, it can actually be *safer,* if you consider the reduction in medical 'interventions' that occur at home. It also won't escape your notice that at home you are more likely to be cared for by a woman (you'd be very unlikely to get a 20-stoneish, bearded midwife, or a male doctor).

is home birth safe?

The Birthplace cohort study compared the safety of births planned in four settings: home, freestanding midwifery units (FMUs), alongside midwifery units (AMUs) and obstetric units (OUs).

The main findings relate to healthy women with straightforward pregnancies that meet the NICE intrapartum (another word for 'in the birthing process') care guideline criteria for a 'low risk' birth.

Key findings

Giving birth is generally very safe

- *For 'low risk' women the incidence of adverse perinatal outcomes (intrapartum stillbirth, early neonatal death, neonatal encephalopathy, meconium aspiration syndrome, and specified birth-related injuries including brachial plexus injury) was low (4.3 events per 1,000 births).*

Midwifery units appear to be safe for the baby and offer benefits for the mother

- *For planned births in freestanding midwifery units and alongside midwifery units there were no significant differences in adverse perinatal outcomes compared with planned birth in an obstetric unit.*
- *Women who planned birth in a midwifery unit had significantly fewer interventions, including substantially fewer intrapartum caesarean sections, and more 'normal births' than women who planned birth in an obstetric unit.*

For women having a second or subsequent baby, home

births and midwifery unit births appear to be safe for the baby and offer benefits for the mother

- *For multiparous women (women having second or subsequent babies), there were no significant differences in adverse perinatal outcomes between planned home or midwifery unit births and planed births in OUs.*
- *For multiparous women, birth in a non-obstetric unit setting significantly and substantially reduced the odds of having an intrapartum caesarean section, instrumental delivery or episiotomy (a cut between the anus and perineum).*

For women having a first baby, a planned home birth increases the risk for the baby

- *For nulliparous women (women having their first baby), there were 9.3 adverse perinatal (occurring during the time of birth) outcome events per 1,000 planned home births, compared with 5.3 per 1,000 births for births planned in obstetric units, and this finding was statistically significant.*

For women having a first baby, there is a fairly high probability of transferring to an obstetric unit during labour or immediately after the birth

- *For nulliparous women, the peripartum (while a woman is in the birthing process) transfer rate was 45% for planned home births, 36% for planned FMU births and 40% for planned AMU births*

For women having a second or subsequent baby, the transfer rate is around 10%

- *For multiparous women, the proportion of women transferred to an OU during labour or immediately after the birth was 12% for planned home births, 9% for planned FMU births and 13% for planned AMU births.*

Chris: OK. I'm still a little concerned about even the idea of her giving birth at home. It's the whole safety thing I guess, not to mention the bloody carpet! Would you say more about why home might be a better place?

Mark: I love your honesty mate, thanks for that. I'm pleased you feel free to express your concerns openly here. By the way, being around other men, talking about our concerns and worries, is an amazing way to prepare for birth. It also fits nicely with the behaviours that stimulate testosterone production, reducing our stress.

I notice that my girlfriend gets so much energy and passion from going out with her friends and talking, talking, talking... Dr Grey observes that blokes will often have two main friendships, and they've got two just in case one dies. We need a back-up, right?

But in answer to your question, let's talk about the impact that the birth environment will have on your lover's hormonal response, focussing on the queen of birth hormones: oxytocin.

Oxytocin is not only important when it comes to birth, it's also the most prominent hormone responsible for sexual climax in women and men. Michel Odent says that sexual climax and birth are one event separated by time; knowing that, we can extrapolate that there is a sense in which the environment that would be suitable for birth is the one that would be best suited for her to experience a body-shaking climax. Now, unless you're into dogging that almost certainly involves privacy, deep intimacy and connection, warmth, a sense of not being observed, not being asked questions. In fact anything that stimulates the neocortex is to be avoided.

To summarise, for great sex it's probably best to be alone and private, and in the natural state of birth the same applies. The commonality between birth and orgasm is profound: both need safety, privacy, intimacy, warmth, a sense of it being something special between the couple, and protection.

Daryce: I don't know about anybody else, but I'm scared about the prospect of not being in control. When I'm panicked, I can come across as an aggressive arse. What can I do about that?

Mark: Your lover will be having a tried and tested hormonal reaction to the birthing process, but so will you; her endocrine responses are complemented by yours. If your lover has evolved to work brilliantly in this way, you have too. For generations our role as men has been to protect her from experiencing feelings of fear.

Feelings of fear, in the early stages of the birthing process, will cause her body to release adrenaline and the family of adrenaline hormones. These hormones are antagonistic to oxytocin, they stop it working.

Daryce: That doesn't make any sense at all to me. You'd have thought that a fear response would be a good thing from an evolutionary perspective?

Mark: Well, imagine you're on the plains of Africa, and she is in the early stages of the birthing process, and suddenly she's attacked. The adrenaline swamps her body so that the birthing process stops and she can flee – remember the four Fs.

Now, this is where the way Daryce's thinking starts to fit in with this mechanism. If she is in the *second* stage of the birthing process when she's attacked, adrenaline causes an expulsive phase of birth. The baby is born quickly, so that she can run away, hopefully carrying the baby.

Joe: So fear can play an important role in childbirth?

Mark: Exactly. In fact, fear definitely does have a place in the birthing process. We hear a lot today about her experiencing no fear while she is giving birth, but actually that's a half-truth. In the early stages of birth, not having any sense of fear is really important and it keeps the process going. In the expulsive phase, or the second stage, giving her space to be with the fear that is naturally occurring inside her facilitates the birth of your child.

I've seen hundreds of women give birth and at a certain time, as her cervix (the opening to her uterus), has opened to about ten centimetres (More pseudo-measurement. Thanks guys! It's not measured with a ruler!), she starts to feel as though she wants to open her bowels. Often a woman will say she desperately needs the toilet; the urge to bear down, like she is passing a massive stool, is very intense and out of her control. This involuntary pushing signals that she's on the home straight; her body is pushing on its own and she has no control over it.

I've watched women as a kind of wave comes over them: suddenly being completely out of control stimulates the four F response and the baby's birth is edging closer. In that moment every cell in your masculine body will cry out . . . FIX HER! But your mission remains the same: connect, be there, be strong, be intimate, offer limited words that reinforce your presence and love. It sounds like melodramatic wank, but this way of being is warrior-like. She will feel your strength, and the 'earth' in you, as the foundations for sacrificial loving fatherhood are laid.

Aiden: God, I'm moved by that! I'm here like that other bloke because my first experience of birth was so difficult. I still get sweaty when I think of it now. I recognise what you just talked about, but that is so difficult to do, because it's difficult to see your partner in pain and fear. I can remember the element of fear; I wanted to think of it in terms of excitement, but really it's painful, it's a bit scary. It was our first time, and I can honestly say I had never experienced anything like the internal pain she was in, and it was difficult to step back. You want to step in and try and offer some kind of comfort.

Mark: Thanks Aiden. I think there is a difference between frantically trying to fix what's going on in the room and doing what you suggested, 'stepping in and offering comfort'. That I think is in keeping with our mission: staying connected, and saying and doing only those things that cement intimate connection with her. It's a deep expression of your love for her and your child.

It is difficult, but it will be easier this time. Preparation, and an understanding of what your purpose is while you are with her, will put your intuitive organic responses to work for you. The insights you get from being here and knowing this information will prepare you like nothing else.

[Note to the reader: We're going to leave the room for a moment or two. I want to tell you a story.]

one couple's story

I want to tell you a story to help explain what doctors and midwives mean when they talk about the 'stages of labour'.

I can't remember exactly when it happened, but I know I had been working in a 'case loading' model for about two years. By 'case loading' I mean that another midwife and I were offering care to a group of about 80 women. The women would see one of us at the start of their pregnancy, then we would stay with them all the way through, including the birthing phase.

The project rocked. Our home birth rate was beyond 18%, women spoke of very high levels of satisfaction, and the service seemed to work (depending on how you measured it). Working this way was very enjoyable, and as a midwife I have never since experienced the same sense of autonomy and stretching of professional competency that the project demanded.

What happened at the time made me feel angry and dismayed, but later, as I reflected on it, I began to see how it exposed the prejudices and narrow-mindedness that can creep up on a group of professionals without them noticing, like a frog being boiled alive as water gradually increases in temperature from cold to hot.

A woman in our caseload had previously experienced a horrendous emergency caesarean section and was requesting a home birth this time. She was being supported by our team; all of the necessary supervision support was given to her and us and the pregnancy passed without event.

Late one evening I was called to her home. She had been having what she thought were early labour tightenings since midday and these had become more intense. 'Please come', she said, 'and see how I'm doing!' She and her partner lived very close to me and although I had a day off the following day I checked in with my colleague and went to see her and the family.

When I arrived, the lights were down, gentle music was playing and she was standing against a pine chest of drawers, rocking gently back and forth, the sway and rhythm of it a little mesmerising, but reassuring.

Her partner started to tell me how the afternoon had gone and when her eyes opened she said she wanted to know how far she had progressed. We talked about her contractions, how long they were lasting, and the frequency between them. I asked whether she was experiencing any pressure in her back passage.

I watched as another tightening ran its rhythmic course and noticed her breathing change, her body take control as she yielded to postures best suited to comfort herself, as the birthing process gripped her. As she grasped his hand I saw the blanched skin of his knuckles and her nail marks left behind.

Having spoken about all these signs of 'labour' she wanted to know how far dilated her cervix was and, having palpated her abdomen and determined the position of the baby, I gently examined her. She had asked if she could stand while I did so and with one of her legs on a small stool we proceeded.

'How far am I?' she pleaded. 'Two centimetres', I replied. Seeing the disappointment in her face I quickly explained that her cervix was paper-thin, the baby's head was very low down and the cervix was tightly applied to it. 'All of these findings suggest that things are progressing well', I said.

We talked for a while as we drank our tea and she seemed encouraged and was keen for me to go home. I explained that first thing the next day I had something planned and that I might not be around.

Her partner asked me to explain what I was feeling for when I did a vaginal examination. I talked about the cervix being thick and hard and round the back of the body, about it softening and thinning and moving to the front of her body and beginning to open, about the baby's head applying pressure to the cervix as it descends, and the feeling of the bulging membranes, like pushing a balloon through a polo-neck shirt. He seemed to be thinking deeply. He thanked me and I went home.

Next day I heard nothing from the couple. I was a little concerned about how they might be doing, so I rang the mobile number I had for them. There was no answer so, assuming that they had been admitted to the maternity unit, I rang the labour ward.

As I expected, that's where the three of them now were. Birth had taken place and although neither my midwifery partner nor I had made it, they sounded very excited about how everything had turned out. I visited them at home that evening and enjoyed the sense of joy, excitement and peace that reigned in the house. Lovely, job done, I thought. I breathed a sigh of contented relief and relaxed.

Two days passed and I was called to see the senior midwife and the risk manager. As I made my way into the maternity unit I was anxious. What had I done wrong? What was it about? Nothing came to mind at all. The previous months had passed without an incident or near-miss. I was anxiously baffled.

The two of them sat, a little stony-faced, around the coffee table in the risk office. Declining coffee, I sat down and asked what the meeting was about. The Senior Midwife explained. 'We've had a complaint about your practice, Mark. The labour ward coordinator two nights ago looked after a woman in your case load. She has raised concerns because when she offered to examine the woman vaginally, her partner said, 'Oh, there's no need for that, she's 9 centimetres dilated. I examined her at home before we came to hospital!' When asked how he knew, and what training he had, he proudly declared, 'Mark taught me'!

They were worried that I had actively taught him to do vaginal examinations. I hadn't, but why not!? The indignation was clear in my managers' voices. 'He examined her!' The unspoken shock at him having put his fingers in 'there'. I couldn't help but chuckle on the inside. I knew they must be aware of where his dick had to have been in order for them to stay in business!

My objective in telling this story is not to say I think it would be good for you to learn how to do vaginal examinations – we already know what your number one mission is when it comes to her giving birth – but to reinforce your growing understanding of the importance of environment when thinking of birth and to give you a guide to the so called stages of labour.

Chris: I think I'm beginning to understand a little more about what is meant by stages of labour. But how will I know when the birthing process has started?

[Note to the reader: When I'm explaining about the stages of the birth process, I show my groups the image below]

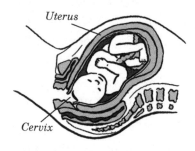

First stage

Tightenings of the uterus cause the cervix to soften and thin so it can dilate and allow the baby's head through.

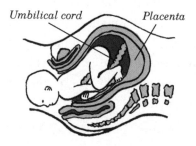

Second stage

This lasts from when your partner's cervix is fully dilated to when the baby is born.

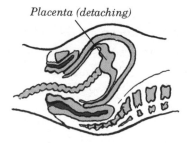

Third stage

Begins when the baby is born and lasts until the placenta is born and when any bleeding that ensues has stopped.

Mark: You've seen the visual guide to the 'stages' of the birth process; let's unpack the stages in a little more detail and as we do I think the signs that things are under way will become apparent. Let's start with the **'latent phase'**. The opening to the uterus is called the cervix, and before the birth process starts it's thick, long and toward the back of a woman's body. Before it begins to open (dilate) it has to soften, thin and come round to the middle of her body.

The latent phase of the birth process is the term for her cervix changing from being thick and hard and toward the back of her body, to coming round to the front and opening to what midwives would call 3 to 4 centimetres. The length of time this takes is undefined and is very variable.

Before the cervix begins its journey to 'full dilation', your lover will almost certainly experience her stomach tightening (contractions). These early tightenings you'll hear called 'Braxton Hicks contractions'.

A Braxton Hicks contraction is a tightening of the uterus that might be uncomfortable; sometimes women say they are painful. They can start from as early as 26 weeks, and although potentially uncomfortable they serve a function.

If you imagine the placenta is like a sponge, when your uterus tightens it squeezes blood around the baby's circulation. So there are two good things about Braxton Hicks: the impact on the baby's circulation, and the fact that they give you and your lover the chance to experience what her uterus feels like when it is tightening.

James: Ah, that's what it was! It happened the other day to my partner, she said it wasn't uncomfortable at all, our baby moved a little more than usual. It was cool to be honest, we got well excited.

Mark: That's very cool indeed James. I hope you got a chance to feel her tummy while it was tight?

James: Yeah, I did. It was quite amazing, it felt very hard indeed. Kind of like a bicep feels flexed. That sounds a little weird...

Mark: I get it mate. Now you know how soft she feels when there are no Braxton Hicks tightenings happening, and you know what one feels like, so you have a reference point for when the birthing process really starts.

Once she gets to 37 weeks these tightenings are almost certainly starting to do something to the cervix, but it's going to happen over time – days and weeks.

There does seem to be a pattern to the latent phase: often a woman will have these tightenings, and they will appear to be coming regularly and getting more intense over time, then as suddenly as they started they go off, disappear for three hours or more, then come back, then go. This pattern can go on, as I've said, for days or even weeks. The tightenings come and go and there are very big gaps in between.

Often you'll hear stories of women who say 'I was in labour for three days'. When viewed as a narrative with no measuring tool applied, it could be said that the birthing process has started, but from a medical perspective what she's describing is the latent phase of labour.

Ben: So at this point no one could answer the question, 'How long is it going to be?'

Mark: That's right. At this point medics and midwives would be waiting for what they call the 'active phase' of the birth process before they begin to make any guess as to how long the process will take.

The **active phase of the birth process** includes the first, second and third stages. The first stage is said to have started when her cervix is 3 to 4 centimetres open. The midwife will talk about her cervix being 'thin': the word for a thin cervix used among birth professionals is 'effaced'.

So with an effaced cervix, 3 to 4 centimetres dilated, with regular uncomfortable tightenings that are coming and going, but not going off for long periods of time, the first stage of the birthing process is said to have started. The length of your partner's birth, according to the doctors and midwives, will be measured from this point, and the first stage will be complete (what medics call complete), when your lover's cervix has reached 'full dilation' and is completely open.

Joe: You haven't mentioned contractions. How many of those will she be getting as this first stage progresses? Are there any clues as to where she is in the process by counting or watching how often they are coming?

Mark: I'll answer Joe's question by first explaining what the 'contractions' are doing to your partner's uterus in this first stage of the birth process. Tightenings of the uterus cause the cervix to soften, thin and come round to the middle of her body, so it can start to open, or dilate, in order to allow the baby's head through.

The uterus is mostly made of muscle, which is tightening up and relaxing. As it tightens, the top part of the uterus thickens, so effectively it's acting like a plunger. The baby only has one way to go, which is down. It's acting like a piston. When we talk about dilation and effacement we're talking about the cervix going from being thick to being thin. It's like pulling a polo-necked jumper on over your head. The top of the polo-neck starts to thin out until it's tightly applied to your head before you pull it over and that's what's happening to the cervix.

As the birthing process continues, the strength, duration and frequency of the tightenings (contractions) will increase. Penny Simkin, in her excellent book, *The Birth Partner* (page 58), suggests that the 'first-time mother' should think about going to the hospital, or settling in for the birth at home (if that's your choice) when she has had between 10 and 12 consecutive contractions that have lasted one minute each, and when the average time between each one is five minutes or less. She goes on to mention that often at this point your lover will be finding it challenging to focus on anything else when the tightenings are present: her breathing will change, her body may begin to move to find a more comfortable position and she may not want or feel able to talk at all.

Daryce: My girlfriend has told me about the 'show' – strange word to use if you ask me! – but how does this 'show' fit in with what you've been saying?

Mark: The words birth professionals use are certainly weird at times! When the cervix starts to soften, thin, move forward and open, it releases a plug of mucus, which has been like a cork or plug that has formed at the opening of the cervix. It is a whitish, mucusy – possibly blood-stained – viscous material, and, as the cervix opens, it is dislodged and comes away. This can happen a week before labour starts, or as the birthing process starts, and some women are not even aware of it at all.

The 'show' coming away is often painless, but some women do say it feels uncomfortable. Because it's often blood-stained she can become anxious and worried about it. If this happens to her, and she is open to being reassured, there is no need to panic. As long as your baby is moving in a rhythm or a pattern that she has become used to, and her 'waters' haven't broken (more on this later), there is no cause for concern. Of course, if she is not happy about anything regarding her baby it's always a good idea to ring her midwife, or the 24-hour contact number you have been given. Mothers' instincts, even before birth, are incredible and shouldn't be ignored.

Ben: Can you say a bit more about the baby moving in a pattern she's used to? There does seem to be a pattern to my baby's activity: loads at night or when she is watching the telly.

Mark: Keeping an 'eye' on your baby's wellbeing is an inside job! I'm pleased you raised this. The only way to truly monitor your baby's health *while he or she is inside your partner,* is through your lover's growing understanding, conscious and otherwise, of the movements that are normal for him/her. The question she should be asking herself is, 'Is my baby's activity level what I'd expect at this point in the day, given my experience to date?'

It's worth mentioning that the position of the placenta can affect how a woman feels the movements of the baby, but his/her movements in the moment are the best way to watch baby's health.

Noah: What about listening to the baby's heartbeat, doesn't that give you more of an idea? I love hearing it! My boss is getting a little pissed off because I've been asking to go to the midwife appointments just so I can hear it.

Mark: These are all great questions. And this one is very important when it comes to your lover enjoying her pregnancy rather than being constantly worried about her baby.

Listening to a baby's heart rate is a nice cosmetic thing and a midwife will do it if you ask, but hearing the baby's heart rate is not monitoring the baby's wellbeing. **The way to monitor a baby's wellbeing is for a woman to be aware of the baby's movements, and patterns of movements.**

Some midwives say that as the baby gets bigger the movements decrease, but that's not the case. They may change in character, but the energy behind the movements will be the same.

At every midwife appointment, you will have heard the midwife ask, 'Have you felt the baby move today? Are the movements feeling like they have always felt?'

Noah: Yeah, every time. It's the first thing she says even before we've sat down!

Mark: That's good to hear, because as I have said it's the most important way of knowing that your baby is doing OK.

In my practice if the movements of the baby have changed to the point where a woman perceives that change, I would say to her, 'Sit down, have a hot or cold drink and gently prod your tummy. If the movements don't resume as you'd expect within ten to fifteen minutes, call that 24-hour number you've been given'.

If you call the hospital and explain the situation you'll

be invited in for something called cardio-topograph monitoring. This machine is able to pick up a reading of your baby's heartbeat and print it out over a 30-minute period, which will give an indication of your baby's health over that interval. I'm going on a bit about this point but it's an important one.

It's really important to me that your lover understands that *she* is the baby's 'monitor of wellbeing'; not the midwife and not the sonicaid (the thing she uses to listen to the baby's heartbeat). Your lover is feeling it from the inside out. I think the way it works is mostly unconscious.

Luca: I don't get that at all, what do you mean unconscious? Surely she has to be aware of the movements to notice them?

Mark: Luca, have you ever met someone, and you can't put your finger on it, but you know that he's a wanker? You just don't like him but you don't have much conscious understanding of why? Often he goes on to act like a wanker and your intuition is confirmed, but sometimes you get it wrong too. Hopefully you did when you met me!

I think that what's going on when you get those 'gut feelings' about strangers, is similar to when she *just knows* that something has changed about her baby's movements. Her unconscious mind is doing its job of letting her conscious mind know.

Going back to the wanker, what happened when you met him? In a split second your unconscious mind started processing, going through everyone you've ever met before, and it gave you a visceral communication in consciousness that said 'Watch out, you've met people like this before and they turned out to be wankers'. It's telling you to *watch out* because, based on a quick summary of everyone you've ever met, this person meets the criteria for a wanker.

I think something similar is happening when a woman is keeping an eye on her baby's movements over time. She is living with her baby's activity day in and day out, and all the time, whether she is consciously aware of it or not, her unconscious mind is pattern-matching.

So when she gets a visceral communication (feeling) that something's not right, even if she's not consciously aware of anything changing, she responds to that and that's the system working well.

Whenever I hear, 'It doesn't feel right, I'm not sure, I'm feeling uncomfortable about this, I'm not sure what it is...', I'm listening very carefully. Even though I might have ruled out everything 'it' might be in my mind based on my experience and training. Just because she can't put her finger on what's troubling her, it definitely does not mean all is well.

Aiden: We had a poor experience of a midwife not taking my girlfriend seriously when she experienced just what you've talked about. What should we have done? We just carried on, and within a few hours Julie was feeling better.

Mark: I'm pleased it all worked out for the best. The truth is that many of the medical professionals I have worked with in the past wouldn't really understand what I have just explained to you. Some do, and others have come to understand through bitter experience when a patient of theirs has had a poor outcome because they ignored her concerns early on.

I have worked with obstetricians (women usually) who get it: often this way of seeing things comes through experience of responding to a woman's seemingly irrational worries, only to find that the woman's intuition was right on the money. The ways of 'knowing' that are based on unconscious pattern recognition seem to underpin all learning.

The medical professional's response is often 'better safe than sorry', but the most important thing to remember is that your lover always 'knows' best, even when you think she doesn't.

Joe: Sorry to add another question, but how will I know when it's time for us to go to hospital, or even ring them? Is it just the timing of the contractions you mentioned earlier?

Mark: The short answer, Joe, is whenever she is not feeling at peace in your own home. When you sense that all that you are doing at home: using a hot bath, dancing to the playlist you developed, massage, TENS machine, moving around freely, focussing techniques (including special ways of breathing), are not helping her to lose herself in the process that is gradually

take action

Think about how you will manage to stay at home as long as you both feel able to (on the grounds that the latent phase might be long, and home is a comfortable environment). It can help to make a list of the things you might do. You might include: a hot bath, use a TENS machine (see later discussion of pain relief), eat and drink, walk around, dance to the music on your play list, massage, watch television... One woman I know made bolognese sauce while in the early stages of the birth process, taking breaks from stirring it as the tightenings got stronger!

beginning to take over her mind and body, no matter what is happening otherwise, if she isn't happy it's time to be somewhere else. It doesn't matter what your mother-in-law says, or the midwife on the phone for that matter. If, after the midwife on the phone has given verbal reassurance and said you don't need to come in yet, your lover still isn't happy with that, just tell the midwife gently but firmly to expect you soon.

Ben: Is it possible to tell the difference between those Braxton Hicks tightenings you mentioned and the kind she will experience when she's in active labour?

Mark: It's true to say that no two women are completely the same when it comes to how their body responds to the birth process. Often, however, there seem to be consistent patterns that can guide us, as we watch her respond to the changing rhythm that her body is beginning to impose on her.

As the birth process unfolds, from what the doctors would call the latent phase of labour to the active phase, the uterine tightenings will last longer, come closer together, and the rhythm of them will be relentless.

James: So when you say they will be relentless, I'm guessing you mean they don't ease off like they might in the latent phase. Are there any signs that the tightenings are the 'real deal', other than frequency and length of time?

Mark: If I'm honest, all the tightenings that a women experiences as she is going through the amazing process of giving birth to another human being are the 'real deal'. One of the less-than-helpful side effects of doctors wanting to measure everything is this insidious focus on 'getting the birth done'. Instead of watching and enjoying the story of your lover's birth unfolding, our tendency is to get involved, in what looks to male eyes like the mechanics of the process. I've gone off on one a bit there, but to answer your question, when I was working in the hospital if a woman phoned in and said that she was having tightenings and they were coming regularly, and did I think she should come into the hospital, I would always wait on the phone for her to have one. A tightening I mean, not the baby itself!

Chris: That's interesting. What were you waiting for?

Mark: I'd be listening to what she was saying for sure; after all, my goal is the same as yours – I want her to feel a deepening sense of connection with me, which will allow the hormones responsible for keeping the mystical birth process rocking and rolling to do their thing.

But I'd also be listening for changes in her breathing, because when a woman gets a tightening in the *active* phase of the birth process, specific things change. One of the first differences you will begin to notice is in the rate, rhythm and depth of her breathing. Talking through a tightening becomes difficult and maybe impossible. If I could see the woman, I would notice that her body posture changes. As the tightening begins to subside and she is able to talk again, I might ask how many of those she is getting in a 10-minute period. If she is having two or three tightenings in a 10-minute period, each lasting up to 45–50 seconds, and she wants a hospital birth, I'd recommend that she make her way gently into the hospital. If she'd planned a home birth it would be a good time to call your midwife.

Aiden: This is bringing back so many memories for me, some of them not so great. I remember Julie becoming very distressed by the intensity of the labour... sorry, I mean the 'birth process'. We rang the hospital and they said to come in, but when we got there, the contractions just stopped!

Chris: Wow, that's exactly what we were talking about earlier. I'm guessing that when she arrived in the hospital, her body

had an 'F's response and it affected that hormone... was it oxymoron or something?

Mark: Ha ha! The hormone is called oxytocin, but it is an oxymoron to think that a strange environment like a hospital is where a woman will feel completely safe so that her hormone factory can keep going full steam.

We've talked about the ideal environment for birth: now let's think about a hospital setting. It's got bright lights, it's full of busy strangers that want you to take your knickers off, and it smells very different from home. All of these factors can provoke the four 'F's and slow the birth process down. In my experience it happens so often I have begun to expect it.

Taking this information and your growing understanding of how all this birth stuff works, should help you to see how important your role is. Doing and saying things that cement a feeling of deep connection between you is critically important at the point you go in to hospital. Staying at home as long as you both can is very important too, but when you get to the hospital you are going to have to step up and be a gentle warrior focussed on maintaining the connection with her.

Be warned, there will be plenty in the hospital environment to distract you from your mission: waiting times, midwives who appear uninterested in your lover's needs, and doctors who push your buttons in multiple ways. Staying focussed on your goal is very important. Ask yourself, do you sense that she is receiving your strength? Is she beginning to lose herself in the intensity of the rhythms of birth? Does she appear to be in another world as the waves of birth are washing over her? The answers to these questions can act as a measure of how well you are doing.

I know I sometimes sound like a New Age, mantra-chanting guru! I don't mean to, but having a mantra isn't a bad idea. What would your mantra be?

Ben: 'Mark is a New Age wank merchant'!

Mark: Thanks very much, Ben! Anyone else?

Joe: I'm thinking, 'Stay connected, speak loving words'.

James: Wouldn't those breathing exercises you mentioned be useful here, given that we'll have practised them beforehand?

Mark: Yeah, for sure. If you have practised the breathing and the mantra together that will work as a kind of 'grounding' trigger. I know, it sounds like more hippy shit. But the truth is, if you do this stuff and it works in your own experience, who cares if it sounds like New Age toss? There's no need to tell anyone about it; just do it, test it in your own experience and if it works, do it. If it doesn't float your boat, do something different.

It has to be said, mind you, that practice means five to 15 minutes of practice every day while she is pregnant until she gives birth. Don't expect to just understand what I'm saying without doing anything about it. That's been one of my biggest learnings in recent years. Just because I understand something, or have read about it, doesn't mean I have the experience of it. Gotta fucking DO IT!

5
COFFEE BREAK: SEX IN PREGNANCY

I'm all for sex in pregnancy, if you hadn't guessed that already. But some blokes (and some women) worry about it. For a little light relief, here's what you need to know.

Have sex as much as you can, as much as she wants. It's great. You should know that the cervix (the neck of the womb) has a really rich blood supply, so if your dick's long enough to reach the cervix and there's any friction, sex might cause a little blood loss. Any blood loss in pregnancy needs to be checked out, so if your lover has blood loss after sex, ring the midwife or the number you've been given for the hospital. Ask your lover if she's happy about the baby's wellbeing, remembering all we've said about her being the only one who really knows how the baby is.

The midwife will ask if the blood loss was post-coital, meaning did your partner bleed after sex? If it happened after sex you can pretty much guarantee it's because there's a little sore or erosion on the cervix that's bled a little. They'll have a look using a speculum.

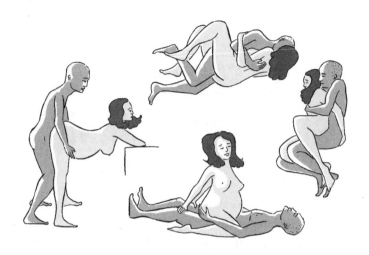

In terms of positions, pregnancy presents a few challenges. Obviously after a few months the missionary position probably isn't going to work very well for her because of the bump, and because she doesn't want to be on her back because of the weight of the baby. There's a major blood vessel, the inferior vena cava, that runs down the left-hand side of the back, and too much weight on it can reduce the blood supply to the baby. The best positions include on her side, kneeling, or her on top. There are some illustrations above of some options you and your partner can explore.

Research was done showing that sperm has prostaglandin in it, which is one of the hormones responsible for starting labour off (although we think the prostaglandin a man produces is different from the prostaglandin that's produced in the woman's pituitary gland). In the old days, when you were talking about how to start labour off, they said to have sex with the idea that the friction of the penis at the cervix caused the pituitary gland to release the hormones responsible for birth. Now we know that semen has prostaglandin in it. But we also know that a woman's orgasmic response is probably more important when it comes to starting labour off, because the family of hormones responsible for birth starting is the same family of hormones responsible for her orgasm. Either way, it's good news about having sex, especially at the end of pregnancy.

There's a bit more on this. One piece of research suggested that male semen was particularly good for starting off labour, but that it was best absorbed through the oral mucosa (mouth). That research was done by a man for sure!

6
THE CONVERSATION CONTINUES

As we get back to the group session, we're going to cover the waters breaking, the effect of posture on the birth process, pain relief, going 'overdue' and induction and augmentation of the birth process. Remember that the conversation will probably spark your interest and send you off to find out more, depending on what you and your partner feel you need to understand as you approach the birthing process together. I don't cover absolutely everything here! But there's loads more information in the resources at the back of the book, and you can use my contact details to get in touch directly if you want to.

Ben: I've got a question about her 'waters breaking'. What's that all about? Will it really destroy the mattress?!

Mark: If you imagine, as the baby's head comes against the cervix, there's a balloon of water in front of their head. And there's water behind their head. That's called the hind water and the fore water is in front of their head, which is down, pressing against the cervix. Often, when the head isn't quite applied to the cervix, that's when you get the waters breaking early. So when this water breaks it often comes with a pop or a gush because it's under pressure. If the waters are going to break before birth starts, often it's because the head isn't making a firm connection with the cervix. So you might get more than what is in front of the baby's head. That can make a mess! It's a good idea to put a towel on the car seat and a pad under the bedsheet in the last few weeks.

Ben: So she'll know when her waters have broken then?

Mark: Not always, they can go with a gush or they can just start leaking. If you think the waters might have broken, you can speak to your midwife or the hospital. They will ask you if you're sure, and if she's flooded the bed, you'll know! But you may not. The amount of mucus that a woman starts to lose at this stage of pregnancy can increase, so she may well feel 'damp', or think she's leaked a little urine. If the baby's well, and your lover's feeling well and has not got a temperature, what I normally suggest is that she puts a fresh pad on (the bag of waters protects the baby against infection, so if it has broken the midwives will want to know that your lover is feeling well and not running a temperature). If the pad is not completely soaked within about an hour, it probably isn't the waters breaking.

Joe: Do the waters going have anything to do with the baby being engaged? That's something I've heard about a lot, but I'm not sure what it means.

Mark: I'm glad you brought up engagement, that's interesting stuff! From about 36 weeks of pregnancy, when the midwife feels your partner's tummy she'll be feeling for where the baby's head is, in relation to the pelvis. So she imagines the baby's head has five parts. Now when the baby's head is above the pelvis we talk about it being free, or ballotable, which means we can move it around. I think that's an old-fashioned word. It's not unusual for a woman having her second baby to have the head free above the pelvis right up until the birth process starts. But in a woman having her first baby, because her muscles are responding differently – more effectively really – the head will drop into the pelvis, and she'll experience what we call 'lightening' at the top of her diaphragm because the baby's moving down. Your partner might say that she can breathe more easily because her lungs are less squished up.

So if we think of the baby's head as having five parts, when I'm feeling the baby's head I'm thinking 'Ah right, three parts of the baby's head are outside the pelvis', so I will write in the notes, 3/5ths palpable, meaning I can feel three parts of the baby's head outside the pelvis. 2/5ths are inside. And that would be 'engaged' really. Engaged is about feeling 3/5ths outside the pelvis, with the rest down and inside the pelvis.

Noah: Once the baby's engaged, does that mean it's in the right position to be born?

Mark: Good question! It reminds me that I want to talk

a bit about positioning of the baby, and the mother. I think it's important for men to know about this. Now if you imagine, when the baby comes down the birth canal, the baby's head comes down into the pelvis and the baby's back rotates uppermost to where the woman's belly button is. So the baby is making a rotation on the way out. Now if a baby starts the birth process with his or her back to the mother's spine, the rotation that the baby has to make is a long one. Does that make sense? Now we live in a society where we sit in bucket chairs, in our cars and at home, and about 35 per cent of women start the birth process with the baby's back to their back. This means that they're more likely to experience back pain and discomfort. The optimum position for the birth process is to have the baby's back uppermost, and not quite in line with the mother's belly button but to the left or to the right. Then, when birth starts, the baby comes down into the birth canal and the rotation is minimal.

What's all this got to do with you? Well, if you understand that this is the case, you can encourage your partner to do exercises that encourage the baby into the best position. Crawling up the stairs, twice a day, on hands and knees. Some midwives say to clean the skirting boards, but she might hit you for saying that! What she's doing is using gravity to help the mechanical process of turning. Squatting helps too. In human history women would have spent a lot more time squatting, to go to the toilet of course but also to work and gather food. It makes sense that squatting and crawling postures would help the baby move down. There's more exercises she can do that can help with positioning and I'll put links in the references.

Chris: This is all good stuff, but I want to know how I can help her with the pain.

Mark: I think the word pain is an interesting one. I think we assume that childbirth is going to be painful; maybe that comes from our reading of the Bible, or maybe it comes from watching reality TV programmes! I'm not suggesting for one minute that the birth process isn't painful for some women, but what I want you to consider is this: we all learnt our mother tongue unconsciously.

Chris: I'm not sure what you're getting at.

Mark: Well, what happened when we were children was that we made associations with words as things were shown to us and labelled, and now those referencing experiences are deep in our unconscious. Every time we hear a word spoken, or see it on a page, it triggers an association, or a memory. So if I'm going to use the word 'pain', immediately you make an association with 'painful experiences'. This happens in a flash and is outside of your awareness, but taps into a whole category of experiences that we categorise as 'pain'.

I've worked with women who have experienced the birth process and the tightenings of the large flat muscle of the uterus, in the context of weight training they have done in the past, as 'just' a muscle tightening. Their experience didn't suggest it should be classified as 'pain'.

So when I talk about 'tightening', I'm inviting a woman to go in a different direction in terms of her meaning-making than when I use the word 'pain'. My experience suggests that some women, when they get hold of this whole understanding, do not perceive their birth experience as painful. Some women even feel that the experience of birthing was orgasmic. This feels a little uncomfortable to talk about, but I had one client who asked if it was ok for her to be given privacy to masturbate during the birth process. She gained a sense of focus, presence and deep satisfaction from being able to climax while giving birth. Most women, when free to vocalise their experience while giving birth, *sound* orgasmic.

We frame our experience through language. The way I *perceive* pain affects the extent to which I *experience* pain. So my advice is, stop watching *One Born Every Minute*! The problem with it is that men and women who have never had a birthing experience are now being shown a fairly limited range of referencing experiences, for theirs. Just for starters, *One Born Every Minute* shows women who have gone into hospital and have agreed to be filmed giving birth. So if you wouldn't agree to be filmed giving birth, you're not like this cohort. And it's hard to see how their experience is relevant to yours at all. We're all far better off allowing ourselves to respond in the moment to what's happening, rather than having an external referencing experience.

Sorry, I've gone off on one again there!

Noah: I understand what you're saying, but last time she was in agony. Can we talk more about the different types of pain relief?

Mark: Yes, let's talk about pharmaceutical pain relief. Now in most hospitals what's on offer is pethidine, which is an opiate. It's an injection, into the deep muscle in the top of the leg. There are some side effects; it slows gastric emptying, so once you have it the midwife won't want you to eat very much because she'll be worried about stomach contents in the unlikely event that your lover needs a caesarean under general anaesthetic. That's very unlikely, because most caesarean sections, even when they're emergencies, now happen under a spinal anaesthetic, which means the woman's awake anyway. Slowed gastric emptying can also cause nausea, and you can have another injection to offset that. Pethidine also crosses the placental barrier, so it does make the baby sleepy, which can delay getting breastfeeding off to a good start in the hour after the birth.

Luca: It doesn't sound that great to be honest.

Mark: It also changes the baby's heartbeat. In some units, once you've had pethidine they want you to have continuous monitoring of the baby's heartbeat for a while to keep an eye on that sleepy trace. If the woman has pethidine, and the baby's born within an hour to an hour and a half, the baby might need an antidote to pethidine, called Narcan, if the baby is slow to breathe.

take action

Make a birth preference list. We talked before about writing your preferred birth story; birth preferences are a little different. Discuss with your partner and answer all the questions you might be asked during birth in your own minds, so that you can point towards a birth preference list. These are preferences about the medical and midwifery decisions that you might need to make, and thinking about them and making a note of them beforehand can be very helpful. The kinds of things to think about are pain relief, skin-to-skin, who cuts the cord and when, whether the baby will have the vitamin K injection at birth, and whether your lover wants a managed or a physiological third stage. (The third stage is the delivery of the placenta after the baby is born; your lover's hormones will usually do a good job of this, just as they did with birth. However, some women have an injection of syntocinon in the thigh after the baby is born that speeds up the contraction of the uterus and the expelling of the placenta. This may be needed if there is additional bleeding, but it does not necessarily have to be given.) You might need to do some research using the resources at the end of the book before you're ready to write your list.

Luca: So you don't think pethidine's much use?

Mark: Having watched women, I would say not. I would say that it works effectively for some and not for others. It can lead to a woman having short-term memory loss as well. So she can feel as though she's not really 'there' for the birth. I've seen it work with women that have been in the latent phase for a long time and haven't got any rest. They have some pethidine, go to sleep and wake up in active labour. But I've rarely seen it work well in the birthing process proper.

James: What about gas and air then?

Mark: Gas and air, or Entonox, is a mixture of nitrous oxide and oxygen that you breathe in through a regulator, off the wall or a cylinder. You can take gas and air throughout the whole of the birthing process – some midwives say you shouldn't take it early on, but really there isn't any cumulative effect. It doesn't cross the placental barrier.

Sometimes women say the mouthpiece tastes of plastic and makes them feel sick, but it's the tubing that's doing that, not the gas and air itself. My feeling is that women can take as much as they want of it, and for as long as they want. There are no real side effects to it.

James: So it's good.

Mark: Yes, I would say beyond a shadow of a doubt. Getting into a rhythm of using it, particularly in conjunction with TENS, can be very effective. Being mobile, using TENS and gas and air, is a really effective combination when it comes to creating an environment where the woman can dip down into herself.

James: And she can control her pain relief herself?

Mark: Yes, she can... What we're doing is we're facilitating a space so that she can lose herself. So that she can have the *quiet mind* she needs to lose herself in the experience.

Chris: What about epidural? I've heard stories of loads of people who haven't been able to have one because it was too late.

Mark: At the moment, 35 per cent of women giving birth in England have an epidural. It's good to know what you think as a couple about the various things that are available. Often a woman will say, don't let me have an epidural even if I ask for one. That doesn't work if women make that decision prior to the experience. Then, as the husband or the partner, you're in the situation of 'What do I do?' because she's begging for one. What I normally suggest – and I got the idea from Dean Beaumont, founder of DaddyNatal – is that you set up some kind of code word and you agree that you will only accept it on the second occasion. The first time she asks you can say 'I hear what you're saying. I'm going to wait now like we decided, and if you ask for it again then I'm taking it that you're making that decision.' That way you're not taking any responsibility for the decision, you're just being the guardian of the coding system.

Daryce: What does an epidural actually involve? We're both a bit squeamish about needles.

Mark: An epidural involves a needle going into the epidural space in the spine. The woman has to sit still, lean forward and curve her spine so that the anaesthetist has access. The needle comes out and a small plastic catheter goes in, which is taped up the woman's back. A small amount of the analgesia or pain relief is dribbled in. In the majority of cases it works perfectly and will stop all sensation from the waist down. Sometimes you get more pain relief on one side of the body than the other. It stays in until after the baby's born; it will usually come out within forty minutes of the baby being born.

Anaesthetists are highly trained, specialist registrars. They're very, very good. But there are occasional side effects to an epidural. In one in a hundred cases, the film around the spinal column can get punctured by the needle, causing what they call a dural tap. This causes leaking of cerebro-spinal fluid, which can lead to a really painful headache. It can be treated with something called a blood patch. Some of your blood is injected into the epidural space and it causes a clot over the hole that seals it up. Anaesthetists will also tell you that there's a slight chance of you being paralysed from the waist down, but they only tell you because we live in a risk management culture. The chances of it happening are ridiculously low.

You do lose sensation in your legs with an epidural, and you do lose any feeling of wanting to push. Now the pelvic floor, when there isn't an epidural, makes a kind of undulating movement. It's the same kind of movement that your gut makes to move food along. Now in theory the undulation helps the passage of the baby's head down the birth canal and out. With an epidural in place that undulation is gone, because the pelvic floor is floppy. Which may well be why there are higher rates of assisted birth with epidurals. So it comes down to pros and cons: the pros are that for most women it's 100% pain relief, the cons are that there's an increased risk of forceps or ventouse (the vacuum suction) being needed to get the baby out.

Joe: So when is it too late for an epidural?

Mark: Some midwives will say it's too late for an epidural. The answer to that is this: ask them 'Will my baby be here in half an hour? Can you tell me my baby will be here within half an hour?' The midwife will say 'There's no way I could possibly tell you that', and you can say 'Thank you. I want to speak to an anaesthetist then'. It's as simple as that. What the midwife is really saying is that by the time she gets the anaesthetist and the epidural is put in and all the rest of it, the baby's going to be here. But she cannot know that for sure.

Siting an epidural is a slightly more difficult procedure if a woman's cervix is fully dilated and she's started bearing down. We talked about the first stage of labour, which is what happens while her cervix is dilating, and the second stage is from when she's fully dilated to when the baby's born. How long that takes depends on who you talk to. When a woman is responding to her body intuitively, and her cervix is fully open, the baby's head pushes on the rectum. So she has a feeling of wanting to open her bowels. A woman left to herself will, at the end of a tightening, just bear down until the tightening passes and the urge subsides again; she'll work like this until the baby's ready to come out. But what you see in hospitals, on the telly, is women being told to put their chin on their chest, hold their breath and push. It's not helpful. It's called the Valsava manoeuvre and it's never appropriate, in my opinion, because if the mother holds her breath it deprives the baby of oxygen. The only way the baby's receiving oxygen is through the mother. When a woman's left to herself the second stage takes longer than if she's directed to push, but that shouldn't be a problem.

In some units they still put an arbitrary time limit on how long the second stage can be. From full dilation to when the baby's born, they might say two hours at most. Some places say an hour! My contention is that when a woman is left to herself, it might take two hours, it might take three hours, but the implications for the baby are not the same as if she were breath-holding.

Ben: The last thing my partner wants is me being an asshole in the birthing room with her, right? So how do I, as a guy, get what me and my partner have agreed we want, past a professional? How do I ask for what's needed without being an asshole and

saying 'I'd like you to note formally on the records that I asked for this and you refused it'?

Mark: It's a tricky one. I think if you try hard to stay present and connected to your lover, and the midwife as we also discussed, asking in the way I suggested, 'Will the baby be here in half an hour?' starts the conversation. She can't say yes or no to that; she doesn't know. If you then follow that up by saying, 'Given that we don't know how long the baby is going to be, I want to speak to an anaesthetist, please', I think most midwives would respond by calling an anaesthetist. Now the anaesthetist may well come in and say, 'I'm sorry but the midwife is saying that the baby is imminent, which raises the risks of putting in an epidural because you have to sit still through a tightening'. Unless the midwife can actually see the baby's head it could well be an hour and a half or two hours, potentially without pain relief, and in my 20 years of experience any decent anaesthetist will put one in given these circumstances.

Chris: Is that pain relief done?

Mark: Not quite. There's water. I have seen many, many women who found that, when they got into a warm bath, the intensity of the birth process seemed to ease. I've also been privileged to watch as women have given birth to their babies in the water. There's no doubt it's a useful tool and some women absolutely love it. In hospital there might only be one or two pool rooms, and there's always a chance there'll be people in there already when you go in, so it's good to have thought about other possibilities too. Some hospitals have large baths that women can use during the birth process, especially earlier on.

One reason your partner might think about a home birth is that it's one way of guaranteeing that she will have access to water, whether a bath, shower or a birth pool that you've bought or hired in advance (there are lots of options). Does the idea of a water birth at home freak you out? If so, find out a little more about it, and listen to what your partner says about it. Bathing in warm water can act as a guide in the early stages of the birthing process; if your partner gets into a bath or pool and the tightenings slow or stop, you'll know she's still in the latent phase and she can continue trying to rest. Being in a birthing pool also enables a woman to be free from too much unnecessary touching by the midwife. It offers a sense of privacy that will cause her ancient hormonal response to flow. In the context of risk, water birth is safe and most midwives will have experience of it, particularly those attending a home birth. There are no side effects from using water, and your partner can get in and out as she wants to in order to be comfortable.

I mustn't forget to mention TENS machines! They're great, but don't let her get in the birth pool with it on! TENS stands for Transcutaneous Electrical Nerve Stimulation. These are electrical pain relief machines, with four pads that go on the woman's back. Sometimes the midwives lend them out, and sometimes you have to hire or buy your own. It's best to get the machine at 35 weeks and practise putting the pads on and turning it up as high as she can bear it, so that when the birthing process starts you can whack the pads on and she can dial it right up. I've seen women get all the way to eight or nine centimetres with just a TENS machine when they've practised ahead of time. But if you get it and only put it on when the birthing process has started you might as well not bother with it. There are a few theories about how it works. One is the gate theory, which suggests that it interrupts the sending of pain messages. Another suggestion is that it causes the brain to release endorphins, natural painkillers. A third theory is that it's just a distraction. I don't care how it works as long as it does! There are no side-effects for mother or baby.

Aiden: Right, I'm feeling like I know a lot more about pain relief. Something that's still bothering me is about the due date; my missus wants a home birth this time and they've said only until one week past the due date. Why do they say that?

Mark: I want to start by saying that due dates don't exist. I know, I know, you hear about them all the time. But the so-called 'due date' is *not* the day your baby is due to come! We talk about a full-term pregnancy being any time from 37 weeks to 42 weeks. A lot of women are given a 'due date', but it's bollocks. It's just 40 weeks from the first day of the last menstrual period. It's not completely arbitrary though, it's also based on a very early scan which is quite a good predictor of when 40 weeks will be, based on gestational age. But the point of the matter is there is no such thing as a due date really. It's just a date with two weeks either side of it that suggests when the baby is most likely to come: an indicator window.

To be honest, post-maturity (or 'going overdue') is made up as well. There's some research that suggests that after 42 weeks the placenta becomes less efficient at supporting the baby through the birth process. So the chances of caesarean section go up quite considerably after 42 weeks. The baby death rate doesn't go up significantly though. So if a woman goes over 42 weeks she isn't necessarily putting herself, or her baby, in danger. If your missus is being told she can't have her home birth, there are conversations she can have with her midwife; ultimately it's her choice where she gives birth, and there are things that can be done, like going in for some monitoring, that will help keep the health professionals happy and reassure everyone that the baby's doing OK. Generally, if a woman's pregnancy goes over 41 weeks, rightly or wrongly the medical professionals will probably start talking about 'induction of labour'.

James: Can we talk more about induction? I've heard that can be really painful.

Mark: Well, let's start by reminding ourselves that we invented the idea of stages of labour, then we forgot we invented them and now we believe in the whole idea completely. We think of birth in terms of a timeframe. Whether you're in hospital or at home, the midwife that you're with will be using these frames of reference, and you're going to have to operate inside them too. From their point of view, active labour is from about four centimetres dilation. The NICE guidelines say that dilation from four to ten centimetres proceeds at no less than half a centimetre an hour, so that's eight hours. And for the second stage of labour, most hospitals will say two hours is enough, so that's ten hours from the beginning of active labour to giving birth. I'm uncomfortable talking about it in these terms, because I think we should be stepping back and looking at birth as a narrative and as a story rather than measurements to be ticked off.

Daryce: So if the stages take longer than that, what will the hospital want to do?

Mark: Let's say the birthing process has started, your partner is four centimetres dilated, her cervix is really thin, she's getting regular tightenings, she's been offered a vaginal examination, then the midwife has waited four hours. When she checks again there doesn't seem to be any sign of the baby coming and when she examines your partner again the cervix is still the same or just slightly more dilated. There's nothing wrong with the baby, the baby seems to be okay. The midwife is going to be concerned that the tightenings are not effective enough for the baby to come. So she's going to suggest a syntocinon infusion. Syntocinon is artificial or synthetic oxytocin. Actually, if a woman's already in labour we're talking about 'augmentation' rather than 'induction' in this scenario.

The brain normally releases oxytocin in dribs and drabs so tightenings vary in intensity. When you've got a syntocinon drip going you will get strong tightenings all the time, one after another. It intensifies the process of birth. This increases the chances of the baby becoming distressed, so if your partner hasn't been being monitored the whole time she will be once the syntocinon is started.

Joe: Can you say something about syntocinon for induction then?

Mark: Syntocinon is also used as part of an induction of labour process, and there are many reasons why your partner might be induced. One of them is post-maturity (going 'overdue') and we've spoken a bit about that.

The induction process involves a vaginal examination being done. We spoke earlier about the cervix being thick and hard and around the back of the body. It now has to be encouraged to soften and come round to the front. And some form of prostaglandin is inserted into a woman's vagina, towards the cervix in order to encourage that process. It depends on the hospital you're in; it could be like a teabag, which is a slow-release prostaglandin, or a tablet, or a gel. After that's been inserted the midwife would wait for about four hours and then, with your partner's permission, examine her again. And if the cervix was open to the point where the waters could be broken, they would ask to do that. There'd then be a further wait and, if birth doesn't start on its own, a syntocinon infusion would be put up which would stimulate tightenings.

I hope you can see from these group discussions how much ground you can cover when members of the group are candid and willing to make themselves vulnerable by asking questions. It's not easy for blokes to do, but your lover will appreciate that you've made the effort. Openness is a quality she loves, and showing it will make a deep connection with her that will lead to a surge of oxytocin. By being willing to learn about your mission, you've already started working on it. Result!

However, remember to follow through on the commitments you have made. A commitment is something you continue to do when the feeling you had when you made the original commitment has gone. That might mean doing something when you don't feel like doing it. At times like this, having a strong masculine friend can offer you the kind of kick up the arse you need. Her feminine essence might respond better to encouragement, but we tend to need challenge to kick-start our engine for change.

I hope that the group session format has been helpful. It may have begun to spark thoughts, raise questions and inspire actions. I want to conclude the chapter by reminding you of your number one goal, throughout her pregnancy and birth, and for the rest of your lives together as lovers and parents:

> *Speak and behave in ways that create a*
> *felt sense of connection with you, in her.*

Over time you will know when you are achieving this goal, and when you are not. If you're not, change how you are speaking and behaving until you are.

This book is a resource. You can use the book itself, the reference list, the bibliography, the video links and my contact details to answer any questions that you still have or that come to you during the pregnancy. But remember, a deep connection with her will probably be best fostered by listening to her concerns and questions as she raises them, and only offering your opinion when prompted by her.

In the next chapter we're going to tackle breastfeeding, as it's the next phase of the hormonal dance that's helped your partner to birth your baby.

7
BREASTFEEDING

In the early chapters of this book I confessed to having always been a fat bloke. For as long as I can remember I have struggled with my weight, although it didn't stop me playing football, rugby and tennis to a good standard. I even played table tennis for the county and cricket for the district.

At my heaviest I weighed 26 stone, felt crap about myself and my body, and was convinced that my girlfriend couldn't possibly want to shag this worn out carcass. Sounds depressed, right? I think I was, to be honest.

But something happened that brought about a complete change in how I managed my eating, and I began to alter my diet and lifestyle. As I write I have lost nine inches round the waist and about 6.5 stone in weight. Like every other massively overweight man I had tried many diets and exercise programmes over the years. Sometimes I lost lots of weight, only to put it back on again.

I know what you're thinking. Relax, I'm not trying to sell you anything. If you're wondering what this has to do with preparing for the birth of your baby, hold on – the punch line is coming.

As well trying every diet under the sun, I had read pretty much everything I could get my hands on about how diets work – or so I thought. Then I discovered the science of metabolism and low carbohydrate diets. In a nutshell, and I have put links in the resource section at the back of the book, when a person begins to reduce their carbohydrate intake to less than 20g of carbs a day, while eating moderate protein and good fats, metabolic changes occur and the body begins to use fatty acids for energy instead of glucose. The early days of the programme were tough, and the metabolic transformation takes up to two weeks to happen, but then I began to experience the effects.

My cravings for carbs disappeared – completely – along with the desire to eat when I wasn't hungry. This was probably for two physiological reasons. Firstly, the body has a store of around 1,500 calories of glucose circulating when carbs are being used as the main source of energy. When fatty acids are being used, the body has thousands of calories available. Secondly, a by-product of fatty acid breakdown is the production of ketone bodies. These are the brain's preferred energy source, and since changing my eating habits, my ability to focus and work for long periods of time has increased. In the past my brain would 'panic' when the glucose in my body was running out. I now rarely feel hungry. I am able to eat wonderfully satisfying foods and lose weight at the same time.

Having learnt about nutrition, and seen the results of the changes I've made, it bemuses me a little, although I shouldn't really be surprised, that there is so much misinformation in the media. The message that exercise is crucial for weight loss is one example. It turns out that it is probably not true. There is little doubt that being fit is a good thing, and exercise increases all round physical and emotional wellbeing, but when it comes to *weight loss* exercise has little impact on whether you lose weight or not. Diet is much more important. However, the processed food industry, which has a vested interest in you not becoming suspicious of the ways it hides sugar in its processed foods, doesn't want you to make the link between the products you buy and your insulin resistance problem. And the industry is enormously powerful. So industry supports messages that encourage you to move more, rather than to eat differently. Because there's more profit for them if you sweat it out on the treadmill and then sate your appetite eating processed foods that are marketed as 'healthy'. Think I'm a conspiracy theorist? There's a huge amount of reading out there on the Internet if you want to know more.

So what's all this got to do with you, your lover and your baby? Or breastfeeding? In this chapter I want to open up the discussion you and your partner will have regarding how to feed your baby. You may already have strong opinions on the subject. I'm not going to go deep into the science of the physiology of lactation (breastfeeding), I simply want to give you a starting point for further reading and thinking. Ultimately, it's a decision that *she* makes – it's her body – and your job is to support her. As with the birthing process itself, and throughout your life together, you need to keep your mission clearly in focus and stay deeply connected. Your support and deep connection will serve you both well as you navigate all the choices parenthood brings.

As we have already discovered, when she feels deeply connected to you her body is stimulated to produce oxytocin. This hormone is not just important for orgasm and birth, it also plays an important role when it comes to breastfeeding.

breasts are not yours

You may have jerked off between them, you may have climaxed over them, but they don't belong to you. They are not even for you. Hey, if your child is to grow to his/her potential they are going to need to drink from them for a long time. *That's* what they're for. You need to understand how milk production works so you can support her as she feeds. No whinging about not being able to hold and suck them! They are not yours. Still, you never know, the taste of her milk might turn you on. Who knows? If not, settle for other kinds of foreplay. Like cleaning the house! (I'm not even joking. Research shows that women are turned on by fathers who pull their weight around the house.)

Just as the big food manufacturers with all the money try to hide the fact that what they are offering us to eat isn't helping us to become fit and healthy, so the big infant milk companies have been doing the same thing for years. It suits them to keep the old chestnut 'breast is best' alive and well, though everyone who works in infant feeding abandoned it long ago because it's unhelpful. Think about it: there's no better way to divide women than to create a 'them and us' culture, putting people under pressure so they feel they have to breastfeed, and making them feel guilty about 'failing', while at the same time offering them products to solve the problems.

It's no coincidence that milk companies own 'sore nipple' cream companies too. Thinking back to how language functions as a meaning-making frame of reference, consider the 'sore nipple' cream adverts. The presupposition is obvious: if you choose to breastfeed you can look forward to having sore nipples. How to undermine breastfeeding without even mentioning it! Perhaps the worst example of language undermining breastfeeding is in the words – often used by well-meaning friends, family and some midwives – 'Are you going to TRY and breastfeed?'. The presupposition is that breastfeeding may not work, may be difficult, and may take a lot of effort. This may be true – and we've all heard from friends and family about their breastfeeding problems – but research shows that most women can overcome the challenges with *support*. A big chunk of that support can come from you.

the risks of not breastfeeding

The risks of not breastfeeding for baby:

- More chest and ear infections
- More likely to have to go to hospital for vomiting and diarrhoea
- More likely to be constipated
- More likely to be obese and to suffer related diseases (eg diabetes)

The risks of not breastfeeding for the mother:

- More likely to have breast and ovarian cancer
- More likely to have heart disease
- More likely to retain weight put on during pregnancy
- Periods restart sooner than if breastfeeding, leading to iron loss (anaemia)
- Any breastfeeding will protect your lover and your baby from these risks, and the longer she breastfeeds for, the longer the protection will last.

Source: NHS. They put it the other way round and talk about the benefits of breastfeeding. I say that breastfeeding's the way we evolved to feed our babies, and that anything else is a risk. Some people find this way of looking at it uncomfortable, but if you read around it I think you'll see it makes sense).

Remember we are mammals, and have been for millions of years. All mammals feed their young milk from breasts or teats. The word mammal actually means that the animal has a mammary gland to produce milk! The use of artificial formula is a *very* very recent phenomenon, and is not as safe as you might think. For one thing, babies fed on 'modern' formula (since, say, the 1970s) are not even in middle age yet. No *long-term* studies have been done. What we do know is that artificial formula changes the body: it alters a baby's gut (breastfed babies' poo is yellow and smells milky, while that of formula fed babies is browner and smellier, more like adult poo) and immune system, making babies more vulnerable to infections. The immune protection that your lover's breastmilk provides cannot be underestimated. Breastfeeding has served us as a species for millions of years of successful evolution, and probably has many more effects on the body than we currently know about – and we know about a lot. If you read about it, or Google the benefits of breastfeeding, you will probably be overwhelmed! Artificial formula can never come close to matching the living fluid that your lover's breasts will produce.

Towards the end of pregnancy, your baby begins to lay down brown fat stores across their back. That brown fat store is there for a reason. A woman will begin to produce prolactin, the milk-producing hormone, from the very beginning of pregnancy, but the hormones that the placenta produces stop prolactin from working.

Some women may leak fluid from their breasts during pregnancy, which can indicate high prolactin levels. In the early days after birth, the placental hormones are flushed out of the body and prolactin can begin its milk-making work: this is why you may hear about the milk 'coming in' on day three or four. In the meantime the newborn baby uses the brown fat stores to keep its blood sugars stable, alongside the colostrum (a thick, rich fluid, packed with anti-infectives, which the mother's breasts produce before the milk 'comes in'.) All the time the baby is taking in colostrum at the breast it is helping to build the mother's future milk supply by stimulating the breasts and the release of prolactin.

At around about 72 hours (three days) after birth, prolactin levels go through the roof at night-time. The baby may go from a pattern of feeding and sleeping, feeding and sleeping, to suddenly wanting to feed regularly through the night. Why? Because the baby is intuitively aware that prolactin is more abundant at night and that the milk supply will be enhanced through those night-time feeds. If you think about when we were hunter-gatherers, when would be the safest time to feed? Through the night, obviously, when things are settled and still.

Milk production is a complete supply and demand system. The more a baby stimulates the breast, the more the breast will produce in terms of milk. Breasts are never completely empty – think of it as like a continuously flowing river, rather than a lake that can be drained and needs time to refill. If the baby has been fed, and wants to feed again in ten minutes, that's fine – there will still be milk available.

Much of what we've discussed about birth applies to breastfeeding too. In the early days, when you get home with your family, your lover's hormones are continuing the birth process and working to produce the milk that will nourish your baby. By focussing on your connection with her, you will support her as she feeds. You may find, as in hospital, that there are challenges that could interrupt the hormonal dance between mother and baby. Conflicting advice from different health workers, too many visitors, your lover's wish to get herself and the household 'back to normal' – these can put a brake on the release of the hormones needed to establish breastfeeding. By staying deeply connected and being a strong presence, you can protect your family's environment in those first crucial days.

Some women – maybe your lover – will worry about whether they've got enough milk to feed the baby in the hours and days after birth. Have a look at the images overleaf. By the age of one month, your baby's stomach is up to 30 times its volume on the day of birth. Understanding that colostrum is low in volume but very concentrated, and that the newborn's stomach is tiny, can help reassure you both. As the days pass, and her milk supply increases, so too does the size of the baby's stomach. It's a dance between the two of them and your support can keep them in time with each other.

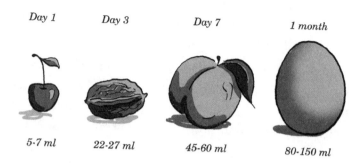

Day 1	Day 3	Day 7	1 month
5-7 ml	22-27 ml	45-60 ml	80-150 ml

As with birth, resist the urge to measure and 'fix' breastfeeding. Read up about what normal breastfeeding looks like. Clue: babies feed frequently, including at night, for several months. The only reliable way to tell whether a baby is getting enough milk is by the nappies: what goes in, must come out! If you are getting plenty of wet and dirty nappies, your lover's breasts are comfortable and your baby is growing then all is well with breastfeeding. Just as confidence in the body's ability to birth a baby is helpful during the birth process, confidence in the body's ability to nourish that baby is helpful after birth. Very few women cannot breastfeed; most can do so with the right support. With you in her corner, your lover has every chance of a successful breastfeeding relationship.

A word about the advice you might get. Many health workers have had lots of training in breastfeeding and know their stuff. Some others don't get it, and still dish out advice that's outdated or plain wrong. Don't be afraid to ask for help, and if you don't like

what goes in...

Keeping an eye on your newborn's poo is a great way to check that they're getting plenty of milk, and if you're supporting your lover by taking charge of the nappy changes, you'll be in the right place to see what's going on. Here's a quick guide to what you're looking for in the first few days:

Day 1: thick, black, smooth poo (looks like Marmite) – this is meconium that begins to be cleared from the baby's gut as they get a few drops of colostrum during the first feeds.

Day 2: very dark green or black/green mix (looks like avocado skin, or plain cooked spinach)

Day 3: greeny-brown, somewhat more textured (looks like curried spinach)

Day 4: browny-yellow with bobbles (looks like grainy French mustard, or crunchy peanut butter)

Day 5: golden yellow with bobbles (looks like grainy English mustard)

An exclusively breastfed baby's poo will look like this for the first few months, until you start offering solid foods at around six months.

the help you get, look for different help! Midwives and breastfeeding supporters should be hands-off when supporting women; touching sends the wrong message. Breastfeeding is something your lover and your baby

MARK HARRIS

learn to do – they need to find their own way (with support). Don't be intimidated by health professionals. Understanding how breastfeeding works will help you tell whether the advice you are getting is helpful.

Some top tips (assuming your lover and your baby are basically healthy):

Don't use nipple shields (if nipples are sore, ask for help to improve the baby's latch (also known as attachment).

Don't wake the baby to get into a 'routine'.

Don't swap breasts after a fixed amount of time, finish the first breast first (baby comes off, or falls asleep), then offer the second if baby wants it.

Don't top-up with formula – if the baby takes formula after a breastfeed, your lover's breasts get less stimulation, and produce less milk. It's a vicious circle and can lead to an early end to breastfeeding.

Don't pressure your partner to express so you can give a bottle, even if you think it will help her out. In the early days she has enough to think about, and some women can breastfeed brilliantly but not produce much milk with a pump. Don't dent her confidence early on. Later on it might be a different story!

Don't worry about how you will bond with the baby if your lover is doing all the feeds. Your role is hugely important and your bond will be strong if you cuddle and care for your baby in other ways. Bathtime, baby massage and carrying the baby in a sling are all great

where to get breastfeeding support

In most hospitals the **midwives** will be able to help your lover and your baby get breastfeeding started. There are **infant feeding advisors** on staff if you need more help. In some hospitals there are **maternity assistants** or **volunteer peer supporters** on post-natal wards who can also offer support. If you give birth at home, or once you come home from hospital, **community midwives** will visit or offer clinics in the early days. Then you'll be allocated a **health visitor**, who should be able to direct you to **breastfeeding groups** or **peer supporters** in the community. **Peer supporters** are other mothers who've breastfed their own children, who've had additional training in supporting breastfeeding. They can offer understanding and support and help with minor challenges, such as poor attachment/'latch', and they can signpost you to more help for other difficulties. They often run **breastfeeding groups** where your lover can meet other mothers with new babies, which can be very reassuring. There's also a **national breastfeeding helpline** staffed by trained breastfeeding counsellors, and organisations like **La Leche League**, the **Association of Breastfeeding Mothers** and the **Breastfeeding Network** which run support groups, online discussion groups and **Facebook** pages and offer great information on their websites. **IBCLCs** (health care professionals who specialise in the clinical management of breastfeeding,) are also a useful source of support or information. There's bound to be something in your area. Details of them all are at the back of the book. If your lover is finding breastfeeding challenging, you can help her to access the support she needs.

ways to get close to your baby.

In the early days, bottles and dummies can get in the way of getting breastfeeding off to a good start so avoid them if you can.

Part of your role in staying connected to your lover and new baby while they get breastfeeding established might include protecting them from Grandmas or other family members who don't understand breastfeeding. It's not their fault; they probably bottle-fed and that's what they know, but don't let them put your lover off her stride.

Understand that breastfeeding is a biological urge: even if it's hard, her body and hormones will be screaming at her to do it. So if she's tired, sore, worried or all of these, support her but don't assume she wants to give up, or that stopping breastfeeding would 'solve it'. Research shows that if women want to breastfeed (and around 81% of women in England start off breastfeeding) but are unable to do so for some reason, then they are at *increased* risk of postnatal depression. The *lowest* rates of depression are among those women who wanted to breastfeed and did. She's going to need you on her side. Remember your mission!

New research done in Australia and Brighton into men's experiences of supporting breastfeeding has suggested that there needs to be a sea-change in the way we look at birth and breastfeeding education for men. The logical conclusion is that there should be tailored, specific educational breastfeeding programmes aimed at men, and that the introduction of such programmes will lead to improved initiation rates and longer duration of breastfeeding, which in turn will improve health outcomes for both individual babies and humanity at large. It's exciting for someone like me who's spent years banging on about getting blokes involved. One place where this has already been tried is in Brazil – there, in an effort to increase breastfeeding rates, they trained postmen to offer advice and support to new mothers on the doorstep! Sounds mad? Maybe so, but as part of a strategy that also set up breastfeeding groups and trained health workers, it worked.

I hope this chapter has shown you that birth is only the beginning; as you embark on parenthood the deep connection you've made with your partner will give you both the foundation you need to parent your children and nurture your family.

THE LAST WORD

We've come a long way together. You now have plenty of information that you can use in the next few months, and, indeed, in the days, weeks, months and years to come.

I have written this book to try to inspire *action*. Just reading it will not change or transform anything: what matters now is the action you take. You might start with actions that don't involve any physical exertion at all: sitting, listening while she talks, and watching as she makes what may seem like disparate connections in her mind. When you invest yourself in creating a deep connection with her, your life together will begin to transform. You are building the foundation that will support you into heroic fatherhood.

Your mission should by now be very clear: do all you can to stimulate oxytocin release in her. This would be a good goal even if she wasn't pregnant; when she is swimming in oxytocin her stress levels are reduced, she is more likely to be content, creatively engaged with life and to radiate beauty. The side effect of all this is that you are more likely to get laid – result!

When it comes to giving birth, oxytocin is crucially important, as we have discussed at some length. It keeps birth buzzing along, and as she connects to you, a bubble of safety is created. All of the actions we have spoken about will begin to bear fruit: your joint slow dance play list, the multiple weekly massages... your understanding of all that's going on around you and the work you have done together will be all the preparation you need to be fully present with her as her body works to birth your baby. These are exciting times indeed.

One cautionary reminder about the birth environment. If you have chosen a hospital birth, you may not be offered much help to maintain the atmosphere of connection and love. You will have to step up into connection warrior mode: resist the impulse to 'fix' the environment if this will distract you or disconnect you from her. You'll know if this is happening – take a deep breath (You have been practising, right?), regroup and focus your energies on her.

I remember hearing one of those American self-help gurus say – shout really – that he was 'IT' today. He had just told the story of his morning routine, and he said that when he sat on the edge of his bed, coming out from his rump was a thick electric cable with a plug on it.

Intrigued? I was too (though I'm pretty sure it was a metaphor). He went on, 'I stand up, breathe deeply, then plug myself in.' At this point he started to shake vigorously as the electric shock stimulated his whole mind and body. He started shouting... 'I AM IT today, I am IT today, there is no one else today, I am all there is.' At first, like me, you could be excused for thinking that this was the narcissistic ranting of a mad man. But then I thought about it. How do I experience the world? It dawned on me that the world I experience is received through my data-receiving instruments, my senses. I receive the data and then make meaning out of it. In fact, I AM IT today. My perceptions of all that is going on around me are completely my OWN. Even when 'things' happen to me, ultimately I get to decide what they mean, to me and for me.

We've reached the end of our time together, and now, as always, YOU ARE IT. Take action, use all the resources the book points you to, get in touch with me if and when you need to. Do something today, now, that will help you move towards the life-enhancing goal of forging a deep, loving and beautiful connection to your lover.

appendix 1
EXERCISES

Breathing exercise

This is a breathing exercise that, if practised regularly, can help you to keep calm and focus yourself during the birth process and at any other time you need it. It builds up gradually. First you take deep breaths, allowing your abdomen to inflate like a balloon. Breathe in through the nose but keep your mouth shut, with the tip of your tongue on the roof of your mouth. Some people explain this exercise in terms of 'chakras'; I don't. But it comes from traditional breathing practices.

On a deep breath in, count to five internally and then breathe out for five. All through the nose with the mouth shut. Do that in the morning for a few days. It's just deep breaths, nothing weird.

If you're going to sit in a chair to do it, allow your spine to be erect. But you can do this standing up; you can do it anywhere. I want you to get to the point where you are focussed on it for five minutes. You can do it while you're shaving if you like – you don't have to be meditating. It's not meditation. It's just a grounding exercise because most of us are not breathing from our diaphragms. If you breathe deep enough, your diaphragm goes down and you feel a bulge in your bollocks. A full sensation in your groin. If you're feeling a sensation in your groin, you're doing it right.

The next part of the exercise is to imagine that you are breathing down your front. You breathe in down your front, then feel the sensation in your groin. For the next part (mouth still shut, tongue on the roof of your mouth) as you exhale, imagine the breath is coming up the back of your head and out through the top of your skull. So you set up a breathing cycle. You get the idea? With practice you'll find it easier to dip into the breathing pattern and become present, even if there is drama going on around you.

I encourage you to do this on a daily basis and to use it all the time, including at work.

Deepening of relaxation exercise

This is an exercise to do with your partner. You can teach your lover some of the techniques you've been learning. Start with the deep breathing outlined above. Then you can add pressure. For example, sit near her and press your hand on the top of her forehead. Say to her something like 'Feel the pressure of my hand on your forehead. Now, as I take my hand away, allow that part of your body to relax and feel the difference'. Then you might put your hand on her cheek and press slightly. Say 'I'm going to release my hands and as I release my hands notice your face relaxing'. Then put your hands on her shoulders and say 'Right, squeeze against my hands, and now, as I take my hands away, experience your shoulders relaxing'. It's a progressive body-relaxing technique, using your own resistance as biofeedback.

This exercise instills a deep sense of relaxation that your lover will be able to access during the birth process. It can affect the discomfort that she's experiencing. It offers her an avenue into the state of mind and body that's useful for the release of hormones for birth. The part of the brain responsible for birth cannot be spoken to and instructed to behave in a certain way. It's below the level of conscious control; it's more like digestion and breathing.

This exercise of biofeedback, using the tension of your arm and your gentle grip, helps her to feel the difference between her muscle being gripped and it relaxing. Tensing against your arm, and then relaxing, paves the way to an altered state for her. The hormones responsible for birth cause an altered state of consciousness in her anyway; so this practice can help naturally occurring opiates to be released in the body during the birth process itself.

Language exercise

Every man (and indeed every human) is constantly in a conversation with himself about life: we call it thinking. This can be quite a challenging idea, if you have never considered that the constant chatter that you have going on inside is a narrative about everything you experience.

This *internal dialogue* is at the heart of the Birthing for Blokes programme. You're host to your unconscious and your conscious. The unconscious is an uncritical thinker and it's constantly battling your consciousness, the part that you think of as you, which is very highly influenced by the unconscious. Once you're aware of all this going on you can make choices and decisions around it. You've been shaped by the sum total of all your experience over the years. How you've responded to that experience has set up patterns – a set of automatic preferences – that are the way you 'see' the world. You react to new experiences by fitting them in to the pattern. What many people don't realise is that by being aware of this process you can alter the patterns of thinking. The first step is becoming an observer of your own thoughts, noticing your internal conversation. You will begin to realise that you have more choice about how you feel and act than you may have once thought.

I have a little trick that I ask men to try for 24 hours or as long as they can bear it. When you speak to your partner, or anyone else, try to hear back, in your mind, the exact words and intonation of the person speaking to you. It doesn't mean analysing what they are saying, just repeating back to yourself the words that they are saying as they are saying them. To stop yourself from

baby's senses in the womb

From 5 weeks

Your baby is responsive to touch

From 7 weeks

Your baby can hear you

By 20 weeks

You may feel the baby moving in response to your gentle touch and the sound of your voice

actually vocalising the words, put the tongue on the roof of your mouth and repeat the words in your mind. Have nothing else on your mind apart from the very words that they're saying to you, as they say them. At the speed they're speaking, say their words back to yourself.

It's an odd experience because when you do it over a period of time, you start hearing your own 'voice' more loudly. My own experience, and that of other people who have tried this, suggests that it brings you 'present'. And the person you are speaking to will feel as if they are really being listened to. That's great, because in the case of your lover that will definitely lead to the release of oxytocin and a deeper connection between you.

Posture mirroring exercise

In this exercise I want you to try on your lover's body

posture, when you're around her while she's relaxed. Try to get a feel for how she's sitting. Then notice how she's breathing.

These are really two separate exercises. Start by spending half an hour with her when she's relaxed, then match her body posture and try it on. When you match body posture you start to get a hint of the other person's state of mind. You get a sense of it. It's not mind-reading or anything like that. It's a way of communicating. Really good communicators almost always mirror body postures when talking to others.

You can follow the posture matching with the breathing. Try to match her breathing and breathe at the same rate, without her noticing that you're doing it. Again, this exercise will deepen the connection between the two of you, without her even being aware of it.

appendix 2
MASSAGE
TECHNIQUES

'Positive touch communicates love and support in pregnancy and labour'

This is an easy to follow step-by-step guide to using simple massage and positive touch in pregnancy and labour. Katie Whitehouse is an expert massage therapist and pregnancy and labour massage instructor. Katie has brought touch into the lives of many parents-to-be through her writing and classes.

The importance of positive touch

Positive touch is vital for our wellbeing. Whether we are a baby, a mother, a child, a middle-aged man or an elderly woman – we all need touch to thrive. Of all our senses, touch is, in a way, the greatest. Our skin is actually the largest organ in our body, yet it is often taken for granted. The benefits of touch, although now well researched, are largely ignored.

This is partly because our basic need for touch is,

ironically, intangible: when we need a drink we feel thirsty, when we need food we feel hungry... but if the need for touch is not satisfied the consequences are less obvious and so they are easily overlooked. However, the consequences of long-term touch deprivation are actually profound.

When we are touch deprived we may experience:
- Insomnia
- Depression
- Aggressive feelings
- Low self-esteem
- Increased stress hormones
- Isolation
- Hyperactivity

When we are touched positively we may experience:
- Better sleep patterns
- Stimulation of endorphins
- Feelings of wellbeing
- Increased self-esteem
- Relaxation
- Ability to relate to others
- Reduced pain

Massaging in pregnancy and labour: positive support and connection

Your relationship with your baby begins long before they are born. By using positive touch during pregnancy you and your partner are sowing the seeds for greater connection with your baby after they are born. There is well documented evidence of how relaxation when you are pregnant benefits you and your baby – massage is the perfect way to achieve this. Using massage in labour involves the father or birth partner in a supportive and positive way. The simple strokes in this section are relaxing and relieving.

Benefits of massage during pregnancy

Pregnancy is a critical time of transition for a couple. There are so many changes going on: physical, emotional, financial... using massage throughout pregnancy is a simple way of helping all parties.

- It relaxes you both
- It is a way for you both to communicate and connect with your unborn baby
- Both father and mother can feel more positively connected with the mother's changing body
- The father can feel more included in the pregnancy
- If practised during pregnancy massage is also likely to be useful in labour

Benefits of massage during labour

- Relaxes you both
- Can help create a pleasant atmosphere in the birthing room
- Stimulates endorphins – the body's natural opiates
- Communicates love, support and reassurance (non-verbally – labour is no time for in-depth discussion!)
- Gives confidence to the father
- Can help with the conservation of energy and

recovery between contractions
- Helps to provide relief from the pain and intensity of contractions.

The best massage oil to use

Your skin absorbs up to 60% of what you put on it – purity and nourishment are really important when choosing what to use, especially when you are pregnant: your skin is under stress and you need to consider your baby too!

When not to massage

Gentle massage is very safe, but there are times when it may be uncomfortable for a woman to receive massage:

- if she has a fever or feels at all unwell
- directly over skin that has sores, cuts, burns, inflammation or infectious rashes
- directly after a large meal

If you are in any doubt whatsoever, consult your GP or midwife.

When to massage

You can massage any time – but the best times are when you know you can let go a bit and forget about the day and outside pressures.

Note: Massage should be soothing and NEVER painful. If it is uncomfortable stop straight away.

GETTING STARTED: 0–16 WEEKS

Getting to grips with the fact that your baby really is growing inside your partner is a big thing. Simply spending some time sitting together – father behind mother with hands overlapping over the mother's lower tummy – can be a good way of beginning to tune in and spending some time being together (all three of you). Keep your hands still. Talking and singing or playing soothing music can be part of this.

Sharing the experience

Massage is good for you both – mother and father! Spend five minutes each, gently massaging each other's scalp, shoulders and neck. Use soothing strokes to calm and gentle squeezing to ease tension. A gentle foot massage is also very relaxing especially at the end of a fraught day.

Most important: Always ask permission to massage.

MASSAGE IN THE SECOND TRIMESTER: WEEKS 16–30

Keep massaging in the same way, but you can follow these guidelines for the tummy massage as your baby grows.

Tummy massage

Stroking over the tummy should be slow and very gentle. Use some oil and skin to skin contact. Try big slow circular movements over the whole belly, and slow long strokes from under the rib cage down towards the hips and groin. Remember this is a chance for you both to tune in with your baby.

MASSAGE IN THE THIRD TRIMESTER AND PRACTISING FOR LABOUR: WEEKS 30–40

Now you can start practising massage techniques that will not only help relieve some of the tensions of later pregnancy, but can also be really useful for labour itself – helping the mother relax and relieving discomfort.

Positions

The ideal is to find a position where the mother's shoulders are in front of her hips. This is a great position to encourage good positioning of your baby in the last trimester and also the best position for labour. It is also important to be able to move your hips and your shoulders. Try these positions:

- On all fours
- Standing and leaning forward onto back of chair
- Sitting on a birthing ball
- Kneeling
- Leaning forward flopped onto pillows or bed

Note: If you tire of one position move to another – try and keep upright and mobile in early labour.

SOOTHING STROKES DURING LABOUR

These strokes are ideal between contractions and help the mother to recover and get some energy for the next contraction.

1. Waterfall

Start slowly, stroking with one relaxed hand from the nape of the neck all the way down to the base of the spine. Keep repeating with alternate hands so that there is a long, continuous, flowing movement.

Tips for fathers: Keep your movements slow and soothing – allow your hands to be completely relaxed and mould to the shape of the mother's body. If you notice her shoulders are tense and pulled up towards her ears then gently stroke them down. Tune in with her breathing and keep your own out breath long and slow as you massage downwards.

2. Hearts

Use both hands – start with hands between the shoulder blades and then stroke up and out over the shoulders. Bring hands towards each other so that they meet at the base of the spine before stroking up and over the shoulders again. This movement traces a heart shape on the mother's back. The heart shape communicates love and support.

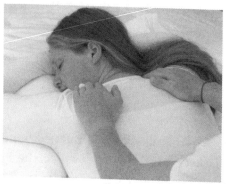

Tips for fathers: You will need to practise these techniques in the last trimester of pregnancy in order for them to be useful in labour. Encourage lots of feedback as to what the mother wants in terms of favourite technique and amount of pressure. You need to build up a language of non-verbal communication (e.g. if she wants more pressure she pushes her body into your hand further; a raised hand means stop etc) as in labour itself conversation is inappropriate and disruptive. Techniques need to be firm but should be relieving, *not* painful.

FIRMER STROKES DURING PREGNANCY AND LABOUR

These strokes are pain-relieving during contractions – you need to apply them wherever contractions are felt, which could be lower back, tops of legs/groin, or tummy.

Lower back massage

The lower back muscles are under great stress towards

the end of pregnancy so massaging them can give great relief from muscle tension. In labour, contractions may well be felt in the lower back/sacrum (the flat bone at the base of the spine) and firm massage here can be very relieving.

1. Sacral circles

Use the heel of one or both hands to apply firm pressure to the sacrum (this is the flat bone at the base of the spine). Use plenty of bodyweight behind this one, and move hand/hands round in a circular or figure of eight movement while maintaining the pressure.

Tips for fathers: Use bodyweight – not arm strength; lean into the massage as much as possible – save your strength as you could be massaging for some time!

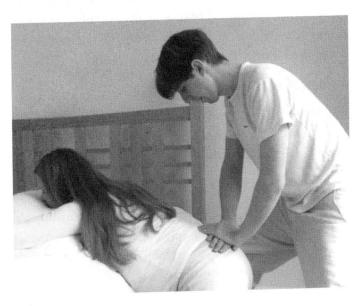

2. Hip kneading

Make a fist with each hand and use to knead deeply into the buttock muscles with the flat part of your fists (or use the heels of your hands). Lean in and allow the pressure to sink through your fists into the muscles. As the contraction intensifies, your fists can be turned backwards and forwards, while leaning in further. This will make the technique deeper and more relieving. You can try working deeply into different areas of the buttock muscles. Be guided by the mother as to the most relieving areas for her, as this will vary from woman to woman.

Tips for fathers: When practising sacral circles and hip kneading in the third trimester, fairly firm pressure can be used – but during a contraction it will need to be very firm (guided of course by the mother's wishes). Adapt the strokes to suit you and your partner – you could use elbows if you have practised a lot.

3. Tops of legs

Use the heels of your hands to sink into the top of the legs – maintain the pressure as you slide your hands down the legs – breathing out.

4. Tummy

Practise this gently during pregnancy. In labour, during a contraction you can apply more pressure as you slide your hands apart. Start with your hands together under the mother's bump. As she breathes

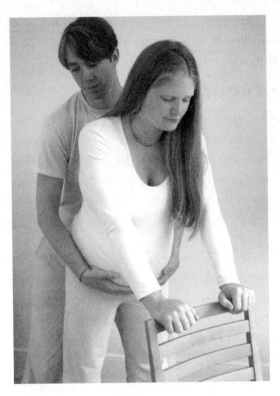

out, slide your hands gently but firmly out towards her sides. Slide your hands in to meet at the centre of her tummy and then slide them back down to the starting point as she breathes in again and repeat as necessary throughout the contraction.

Other ideas and tips

Whilst it is best to keep shoulders in front of hips during pregnancy and upright and mobile in labour, there may be times when she needs to rest. Try a side-lying position with her uppermost leg bent and supported on pillows. It has been found that lying on the left side is ideal for foetal positioning (i.e. to help the baby move into the best position for birth).

Foot and hand massage

If the mother needs to be monitored, or has an epidural, a foot, hand or shoulder massage can be very reassuring. The most important thing is that the mother is comfortable and as relaxed as possible. Massage can help bring some of your home environment into a labour room in a hospital – especially if you have practised!

Tips for stage one

This stage begins with regular contractions, building up in strength, duration, and frequency, getting closer together as the mother's cervix dilates from 0–10cm to allow the baby's head to pass through into the birth canal. The following may be helpful:

- Using massage for relaxation and to ease discomfort
- Staying upright and mobile with shoulders in front of hips
- Keeping hips moving
- Being held and supported
- Deep warm baths (once labour is established)
- Breathing – focus on the out breath during contractions – make it long and drawn out

Encourage her to listen to and trust her instincts. She can move into the position that feels right for her and change position as she feels necessary – and make any noises that feel helpful to her. Above all she can try to keep an open mind and try and stay as calm as possible.

Tips for transition

This is when the cervix is almost fully dilated and she is building up to stage two (the actual birth). She may feel a sudden change of mood, or a state of altered being; possibly a need to be left alone. The following may be helpful:

- Inhaling scented oils
- Kneeling or leaning forward
- Sips of water
- Cool water on a flannel to mop her brow
- Making long, drawn-out noises
- Focussing on the slow outbreath
- Sacral circles

Once your baby is born

Try to ensure that your partner, or you if she cannot, has prolonged skin-to-skin contact with your baby as soon as possible after they are born.

BRINGING TOUCH INTO EVERYDAY LIFE

We live in a touch-deprived and busy world. Whether we were massaged as babies or not, and whether or not we massaged our own babies, in my experience it is never too late to start. It can be very simple to bring massage and positive touch into our everyday lives. With the clear boundary that touch must always be wanted and that we should be able to say no to unwanted touch, I believe that a profound difference could be made very simply. As well as massaging your baby you could also try:

- Offering someone you know who is elderly and possibly rarely touched (maybe your own parent or grandparent) a hand massage next time you visit. It is unintrusive but really relaxing and easy to carry on talking while you do it.
- Offering your children a very gentle soothing back massage before they go to sleep. Simply stroke downwards from head/neck to the base of their spine. You can do this over their pyjamas so they are able to stay relaxed and drop off to sleep.
- Offering your partner a five-minute neck and shoulder massage this evening.

Katie Whitehouse is the founder of Vital Touch, who make the Natalia range of oils for use in pregnancy and labour. The prenatal body and bath oil is cold-pressed organic sunflower and rich avocado oil with an appropriate dilution of organic roman chamomile, lavender and sweet orange to relax and warm tense muscles and relieve stress. The labour massage oil is organic sunflower oil with a supportive blend of clary sage, jasmine and uplifting bergamot. Natalia instant energiser can be used to inhale during labour. For more details see www.vitaltouch.com.

FURTHER READING AND RESOURCES

This is a big resource section. Everything in here has informed the writing of this book. I love the way that reading one book can stimulate learning, a desire to take paths that you never anticipated taking, ending up in unknown places that serve to deepen your appreciation of life in general, whilst broadening your understanding of the original subject.

Enjoy. And, if something here prompts you, I repeat that I am happy for you to make contact with me personally.

Books

Andreas, C. (1996) *Core Transformation: Reaching the Wellspring Within*. United States: Real People Press

Bandler, R. (2008) *Get the Life You Want*. United States: Health Communications

Bandler, R. (2008) *Richard Bandler's Guide to Trance-formation*. United States: Health Communications

Bandler, R., Grinder, J. (1990) *Frogs into Princes: Neuro Linguistic Programming*. United Kingdom: Eden Grove Editions

Barnes, B., Badley, S.G. (1990) *Planning for a Healthy Baby*, United Kingdom: Ebury

Baron-Cohen, S. (2012) *The Essential Difference: Men, Women and the Extreme Male Brain*. United Kingdom: Penguin Books

Beaumont, D. (2013) *The Expectant Dad's Handbook: All You Need to Know about Pregnancy, Birth and Beyond*. United Kingdom: Vermilion

Bourgeault, C. and Moore, T. (2003) *The Wisdom Way of Knowing: Reclaiming an Ancient Tradition to Awaken the Heart*. United States: Wiley, John & Sons, Incorporated

Brizendine, L. (2008) *The Female Brain*. United Kingdom: Bantam Books

—— (2011) *The Male Brain*. United Kingdom: Bantam Books

Buckley, S. (2009) *Gentle Birth, Gentle Mothering: A Doctor's Guide to Natural Childbirth and Gentle Early Parenting Choices*. United States: Celestial Arts

Byrom, S. and Downe, S. (eds.) (2014) *The Roar Behind the Silence: Why Kindness, Compassion and Respect Matter in Maternity Care*. United Kingdom: Pinter & Martin

Churchill, H. and Savage, W. (2008) *How to avoid an unnecessary Caesarean: a Handbook for Women Who Want a Natural Birth*. United Kingdom: Pinter & Martin

Darwin, C. and Wallace, J. (1998) *The Origin of Species*. United Kingdom: NTC/Contemporary Publishing Company

Deida, D. (1997) *It's a Guy Thing: an Owner's Manual for Women*. United States: Health Communications

—— (2002) *Naked Buddhism: 39 Ways to Free Your Heart and Awaken to Now*. United States: Plexus

—— (2004) *The Way Of The Superior Man: A Spiritual Guide to Mastering the Challenges of Woman, Work, and Sexual Desire*. United States: Sounds True

—— (2005) *Dear Lover: A Woman's Guide To Men, Sex, And Love's Deepest Bliss*. United States: Sounds True

Eicher, J. (1993) *Making the Message Clear: How to Master the Business Communication Tools that Direct Productivity, Excellence and Power*. United States: Grinder, Delozier & Associates

England, P. and Horowitz, R. (1998) *Birthing From Within*. United States: Partera Press

Ekman, P. (2008) *Emotional Awareness: Overcoming the Obstacles to Psychological Balance and Compassion*. United Kingdom: Times Books

—— with Freisen, W.V. (2007) *Unmasking the Face*. Malor United States: Malor Books

—— (2003) *Emotions Revealed: Recognizing Faces and Feelings to Improve Communication and Emotional Life*. United Kingdom: Times Books

—— (1985) *Telling Lies: Clues to Deceit in the Marketplace, Politics, and Marriage*. United States: W. W. Norton & Company

—— with Rosenberg, E. L. (1998) *What the Face Reveals*. United Kingdom: Oxford University Press

—— with Davidson, R. (1994) *The Nature of Emotion: Fundamental Questions*. United Kingdom: Oxford University

—— (1974) *Darwin and Facial Expression: A Century of Research in Review*. United Kingdom: Academic Press Inc.

—— (1993) *Facial Action Coding System / Investigator's Guide Part I*. United States: Consulting Psychologists Press

—— (1991) *Why Kids Lie: How Parents Can Encourage Truthfulness*. United States: Penguin

—— with Scherer, K.R., (1992) *Handbook of Methods in Nonverbal Behavior Research*. United Kingdom: Cambridge University Press

—— (1980) *Face of Man: Expressions of Universal Emotions in a New Guinea Village.* United States: Garland Publishing

—— with Friesen W.V. and Ellsworth, P. (1972) *Emotion in the Human Face: Guidelines for Research and an Integraion of Findings.* United Kingdom: Pergamon.

—— (1999) *Handbook of Cognition and Emotion.* United Kingdom: John Wiley & Sons, Ltd.

Evans, K. (2014) *Bump. How to Make, Grow and Birth a Baby.* United Kingdom: Myriad Editions

—— (2008) *The Food of Love: Your Formula for Successful Breastfeeding.* United Kingdom: Myriad Editions

Fine, C. (2011) *Delusions of Gender: The Real Science Behind Sex Differences.* London: Icon Books

Fletcher, S. (2014) *Mindful Hypnobirthing: Hypnosis and mindfulness techniques for a calm and confident birth.* United Kingdom: Vermilion

Gaskin, I. M. (2008) *Ina May's Guide to Childbirth.* United Kingdom: Vermilion

Gerhardt, S. (2004) *Why Love Matters.* United Kingdom: Routledge

Gonzalez, C. (2014) *Breastfeeding Made Easy: A Gift for Life for You and Your Baby.* United Kingdom: Pinter & Martin

González, C. (2012) *Kiss me!: How to Raise Your Children with Love.* United Kingdom: Pinter & Martin

Gordon, D.C. (1978) *Therapeutic Metaphors: Helping Others Through the Looking Glass.* United States: Meta Publications

Gosling, S. (2008) *Snoop: the Secret Language of Everyday Things.* United Kingdom: Profile Books

Gray, J. (2003) *Mars And Venus In The Bedroom: A Guide to Lasting Romance and Passion.* United Kingdom: Vermilion

Grayson, H. (2004) *Mindful Loving*. United States: Gotham

Hall, M. L. (2001) *The Spirit of NLP*. United Kingdom: Crown House Publishing

Hanssen, H. (2013) *Baby Management for Men: A Very Practical Guide*. United Kingdom: Pinter & Martin

Hazard, L. (2010) *The Father's Home Birth Handbook*. United Kingdom: Pinter & Martin

Heli, S. (2013) *Confident Birth*. United Kingdom: Pinter & Martin

Hyatt, C. and Wilson, R. A. (1992) *To Lie is Human: Not Getting Caught is Divine*. United States: New Falcon Publications

Jory, M. (2007) *Beyond Freedom: Talks with Sri Nisargadatta Maharaj*. United States: Yogi Impressions Books Pvt. Ltd.

Jowitt, M. (2014) *Dynamic Positions in Birth: A Fresh Look at How Women's Bodies Work in Labour*. United Kingdom: Pinter & Martin

Kemeny, N. (2014) *Nurturing New Families*. United Kingdom: Pinter & Martin

Kitzinger, S. (2004) *The New Experience of Childbirth*. United Kingdom: Orion

Kitzinger, S. (2015) *A Passion for Birth: My Life: Anthropology, Family and Feminism*. United Kingdom: Pinter & Martin

Klein, J. and Edwards, E. (2006) *I Am*. United Kingdom: Non-Duality Press

Laborde, G. (2003) *Influencing with Integrity: Management Skills for Communication and Negotiation*. Revised Edition. United Kingdom: Crown House Publishing

La Leche League International (2014) *Sweet Sleep*. United Kingdom: Pinter & Martin

—— (2010) *The Womanly Art of Breastfeeding.* United Kingdom: Pinter & Martin

Leboyer, F. (1997) *Birth Without Violence.* United Kingdom: Pinter & Martin

Marshall, H., Klaus, M.H., Kennel, J.H. and Klaus, P.H. (2012) *The Doula Book.* United States: Da Capo Lifelong Books

McMahon, M. (2015) *Why Doulas Matter.* United Kingdom: Pinter & Martin

Odent, M. (1994) *Birth Reborn: What Childbirth Should Be.* United Kingdom: Souvenir Press

—— (2009) *The Functions of the Orgasms: the Highways to Transcendence.* London: Pinter & Martin

Palmer, G. (2009) *The Politics of Breastfeeding: When Breasts Are Bad for Business.* United Kingdom: Pinter & Martin

Rhinehart, L. (2000) *The Book of the Die: [A Handbook of Dice Living].* United Kingdom: HarperCollins Publishers

Simkin, P. (2013) *The Birth Partner: A Complete Guide to Childbirth for Dads, Doulas, and Other Labor Companions.* United States: Harvard Common Press

Stadlen, N. (2005) *What Mothers Do – Especially When It Looks Like Nothing.* United Kingdom: Piatkus

—— (2011) *How Mothers Love.* United Kingdom: Piatkus

Stockton, A. (2010) *Gentle Birth Companions: Doulas Serving Humanity.* United Kingdom: McCubbington Press

—— (2009) *Birth Space, Safe Place: Emotional Well-Being Through Pregnancy and Birth.* United Kingdom: Findhorn Press

Sundin, J. (2008) *Birth Skills: Proven Pain-Management Techniques for your Labour and Birth.* United Kingdom: Vermilion

Sutton, J. (2001) *Let Birth be Born Again! Rediscovering & Reclaiming our Midwifery Heritage.* United Kingdom: Birth Concepts

Taubes, G. (2012) *Why We Get Fat: And What to Do About It* United States: Knopf Doubleday Publishing Group

Taylor, E. (2014) *Becoming Us: 8 Steps to Grow a Family that Thrives.* Australia: Three Turtles Press

Trevathan, W. (2010) *Ancient Bodies, Modern Lives: How Evolution has Shaped Women's Health.* United Kingdom: Oxford University Press

Walsh, D. (2007) *Evidence-Based Care for Normal Labour and Birth: A Guide for Midwives.* United Kingdom: Routledge

Welford, H. (2011) *Successful Infant Feeding: Ensuring your Baby Thrives on the Breast or Bottle.* United Kingdom: Carroll & Brown

Westman, E.C., Phinney, S.D. and Volek, J. (2010) *New Atkins for a New You: The Ultimate Diet for Shedding Weight and Feeling Great.* United Kingdom: Ebury Press

Wilson, R. A. (1990) *Quantum Psychology: How Brain Software Programs You and Your World.* United States: New Falcon Publications

Woodsmall, M. and Woodsmall, W. (1998) *People Pattern Power: P3: The Nine Keys to Business Success.* United States: Next Step Press

Websites

Doula UK articles on what a doula is
doula.org.uk/content/what-doula
doula.org.uk/content/what-do-doulas-do

The origins of the doula – a global perspective
adelastockton.co.uk

A round up on the research on doula support
evidencebasedbirth.com/the-evidence-for-doulas

Pre-conception and conception information and support
foresight-preconception.org.uk

Finding a doula in your area
doula.org.uk/find-a-doula

Honouring the last days of pregnancy
mothering.com/articles/the-last-days-of-pregnancya-place-of-in-between

Evidence around induction of labour
sarawickham.com/tag/induction

Maternity and human rights
birthrights.org.uk
humanrightsinchildbirth.com
jesusaricoy.blogspot.co.uk/2013/11/the-roses-revolutionpeaceful-movement.html
aims.org.uk

Positive peer support
positivebirthmovement.org
tellmeagoodbirthstory.com

Childbirth preparation
ahaparenting.com
bellybelly.com.au/birth/birth-plan-can-you-planbirth

Comfort and control during childbirth
birthunplugged.blogspot.co.uk/2010/11/traditional-
birthsecrets-rebozo.html
natalhypnotherapy.co.uk
mindfulmamma.co.uk
thewisehippo.com
thehypnobirthingcentre.co.uk
activebirthcentre.com
birthlight.co.uk
nct.org.uk/courses/antenatal/antenatal-services/relax-
stretch-and-breathe-nct-yoga-pregnancy

Inspiration, information and choice
aims.org.uk AIMS booklets, especially *Am I allowed*
which.co.uk/birth-choice
anthrodoula.blogspot.co.uk/2011/06/informed-choice-
and-brain-acronym.html
pregnancy.com.au/birth-choices/homebirth/out-of-the-
laboratory-back-to-the-darkened-room.shtml
sarahbuckley.com/articles

Second stage of labour and the immediate postnatal period
thebirthpause.com
bellybelly.com.au/baby/why-its-best-to-avoid-putting-
a-hat-on-your-newborn-baby

Third stage of labour – birthing your placenta
midwifethinking.com/2010/08/26/the-placenta-
essential-resuscitation-equipment

kangaroomothercare.com
sarahbuckley.com/leaving-well-alone-a-natural-
approach-to-the-third-stage-of-labour
aims.org.uk/pubs3.htm
placentanetwork.com/research-and-articles/placenta-
the-forgotten-chakra-by-robin-lim

The science of infant sleep
isisonline.org.uk
babymanualnotincluded.com

Postnatal support
doublehelpingdoulas.co.uk/blog
thebirthhub.co.uk/closing-bones
bellybelly.com.au/post-natal/birth-release-ceremony-
healing-when-your-birth-didnt-go-to-plan
oneplusone.org.uk/content_topic/becoming-aparent/
common-problems-for-new-parents

Feeding – issues, politics and advocacy
who.int/nutrition/publications/
infantfeeding/9241541601/en/
analyticalarmadillo.co.uk

Unbiased information on breastmilk substitutes
firststepsnutrition.org/newpages/infants/infant_
feeding_infant_milks_UK.html
babymilkaction.org

Feeding support
kellymom.com
abm.me.uk
breastfeedingnetwork.org.uk

laleche.org.uk
nct.org.uk/parenting/feeding

The science and psychology of parenting
normalfed.com/onion
analyticalarmadillo.co.uk

Fathers/Partners
daddynatal.co.uk
birthingawareness.com/birthing-for-blokes
fatherstobe.org
fatherhoodinstitute.org

Unassisted birth
aims.org.uk/Journal/Vol19No3/itIsIllegal.htm
birthrights.org.uk/library/factsheets/UnassistedBirth.
   pdf
unassistedchildbirth.com

Special care
parenting.com/article/leaving-baby-behind

Birth trauma and mental health support
birthtraumaassociation.org.uk
pandasfoundation.org.uk
petalscharity.org

Losing a child
uk-sands.org

Debriefing
birchtreebeginnings.co.uk/birth-debriefing/

Becoming a doula
doula.org.uk/content/journey-being-doula

doula.org.uk/content/becoming-doula

Doula UK approved training courses
doula.org.uk/content/list-doula-uk-recognised-courses

Maddie McMahon's course and websites
developingdoulas.co.uk

thebirthhub.co.uk

maddiemcmahon.com

Michel Odent doula course
paramanadoula.com/index.html

Living with a doula and doulas reflect on their role
wonderfullymadebelliesandbabies.blogspot.
   co.uk/2014/03/my-wifes-doula.html

anthrodoula.blogspot.co.uk/2011/09/being-doula-is-
   hard.html

jodithedoula.com/2013/03/02/no-free-births

northeastdoulas.com/blog/becoming-doulas-husband

Videos

www.birthing4blokes.com
Here you will find video links for the following subjects. You will notice, having read the book, that the language in the titles of some of these videos is not always the best that it could be in terms of your meaning-making, but hey ho, it's the language you will probably hear while she is pregnant.

When you go to the website you will find tabs for each of these subjects, and some commentary:

Induction of labour

What is post-maturity

The stages of labour

Staying at home as long as possible

Home birth

Pain relief options

When to call the midwife

Tests available in pregnancy

Why low carbohydrate diets work

Dr John Grey

There is more stuff on the page too, so enjoy, and remember you can call or email me anytime.

Breastfeeding support

National Breastfeeding Helpline 0300 100 0212
nationalbreastfeedinghelpline.org.uk

La Leche League helpline 0845 120 2918
laleche.org.uk/content/telephone-helpline

The Association of Breastfeeding Mothers
0300 330 5453 abm.me.uk

The Breastfeeding Network Drugs In Breastmilk
Helpline 0844 412 4665

ACKNOWLEDGEMENTS

A life is not lived alone. It sounds cheesy, but without my family and friends my life would not be the extravagant adventure it is.

The men who I love are all acknowledged in the conversation section of the book. Thank you Ben, Joe and Daryce, my sons; the truth is, I'd choose you as friends. I love you.

Chris, brothers till we die. Thank you.

My daughters Amy, Laura, and Abbi: you have all become amazing mothers. Diane would be proud of you.

Trez, James and Bella, I love you. Thank you for accepting me into your family.

Trez, nearly crying (usual for me) as I think about the countless different ways that your love for me inspires a deep sense of gratitude.

It's difficult to put into words the debt that I owe to Susan Last. You have been a constant source of encouragement and grace, your honest feedback and brilliant work makes the book what it has become. Thank you.

Pinter & Martin, my publishers, I owe you a big thank you. I wasn't really thinking of writing anything until your faith in what I had to say stirred something in me that resulted in this book.

INDEX

fight, flight, freeze and
'reproduction' (the four
Fs) 74, 87, 88, 108
'fixing', men's tendency
towards
and the birth process
55, 69–70, 72–3, 75–6,
88
and breastfeeding 144,
148
comforting vs. 'fixing'
88–9
and the loving
connection between
partners 48, 53
and testosterone 79
food industry 137, 138
forceps/ ventouse births
125
formula feeding 139–41,
146

gas and air 122–3
goal-driven, men as 53,
75–6
Grey, John 60–1, 73, 77

heartbeat, listening to
baby's 100–1
home
best place for early
stages of birth process
34, 105–6
home births 80–6, 128,
129–30
hormones
and breastfeeding 141

and 'energy' 60
gender differences 54,
59–61, 76–7, 79, 86
and the limbic system
28
men's hormonal
response to birth 86
oestrogen 61, 63, 79
and orgasm 32, 53,
85–6
prolactin 141–2
prostaglandin 112–13,
132
see also adrenaline;
oxytocin; testosterone
hospital births
creating a suitable
birth space 33–4, 108
safety of 80–4
and 'warrior' mode 151
when to go in for 98–9,
104–7
housework
as foreplay 53, 143
and the loving
connection 47
and oxytocin 53

induction of birth process
130–3
instincts, maternal 100–4
internal dialogue 156
intimacy within the birth
room 71, 73, 86, 88
see also connection,
importance of

Korbisky, Alfred 44

lactation consultants *see* breastfeeding support
language exercise 155–7
latent phase of birth process 34, 95–7, 104–6
'lightening' 116
lighting, dim 31, 33–4
limbic system of brain 27–8, 29–30, 41, 74–5
listening, importance of 70, 72–3, 134
loving connection *see* connection, importance of

'masculine presence', need for 59–60
masculinity of the birth process 53, 54–6, 75–6, 78, 106
massage 31–2, 159–72
maternal instincts 100–4
Mead, Margaret 40
meaning-making brains 28, 37, 41–2, 44, 49, 74
measurement, in the birth process 75–6, 79, 106, 126, 131
medicalisation of birth 29, 54–6, 75–6
mental preparation 65–6
midwives
    caring for your midwives 66–7
    case loading 89

connection with 48, 66, 127
    midwife-led units 81–4
    oxytocin levels of 66
mirroring 50–1, 157–8
mothering a partner 53, 55
movements, baby's 100–2
multi-level communication 38–51, 66, 155–7
music playlists 33, 35

narratives/ story 79–80, 106, 131
neocortex of brain 27–30, 41–2, 59, 74, 86
NICE guidelines 131
nutrition 136–7

Odent, Michel 30–1, 52, 54–5, 85
oestrogen 61, 63, 79
One Born Every Minute (avoiding) 119
orgasm
    and birth 30–1, 53, 85–6, 119
    and massage 31–2
    and oxytocin 32, 53, 85–6
    in pregnancy 31–2
    starting birth process off 113
overdue babies 130
oxytocin
    and adrenaline 30, 86
    breastfeeding 31, 138